NEUROSCIENCE OF COMMUNICATION

Singular Textbook Series
Editor: M. N. Hegde, Ph.D.

Applied Phonetics: The Sounds of American English
by Harold T. Edwards, Ph.D.

Applied Phonetics Workbook: A Systematic Approach to Phonetic Transcription
by Harold T. Edwards, Ph.D., and Alvin L. Gregg, Ph.D.

Applied Phonetics Instructor's Manual
by Harold T. Edwards

Assessment in Speech-Language Pathology: A Resource Manual
by Kenneth G. Shipley, Ph.D., and Julie G. McAfee, M.A.

Child Phonology
by Ken Bleile, Ph.D.

Clinical Methods and Practicum in Speech-Language Pathology
by M. N. Hegde, Ph.D., and Deborah Davis, M.S.

Clinical Methods and Practicum in Audiology
by Ben R. Kelly, Ph.D., Deborah Davis, M.S., and M. N. Hegde, Ph.D.

Clinical Speech and Voice Measurement: Laboratory Exercises
by Robert F. Orlikoff, Ph.D., and Ronald J. Baken, Ph.D.

Clinical Speech and Voice Measurement: Instructor's Manual
by Robert F. Orlikoff, Ph.D., and Ronald J. Baken, Ph.D.

A Coursebook on Scientific and Professional Writing in Speech-Language Pathology
by M. N. Hegde, Ph.D.

Diagnosis in Speech-Language Pathology
edited by J. Bruce Tomblin, Ph.D., D. C. Spriesterbach, Ph.D., and Hughlett Morris, Ph.D.

Introduction to Clinical Research in Communication Disorders
by Mary Pannbaker, Ph.D., and Grace Middleton, Ed.D.

Introduction to Communication Sciences and Disorders
edited by Fred D. Minifie, Ph.D.

Student Workbook for Introduction to Communication Sciences and Disorders
by Fred D. Minifie, Ph.D., with Carolyn R. Carter and Jason L. Smith

Instructor's Manual for Introduction to Communication Sciences and Disorders
by Fred D. Minifie, Ph.D.

Language and Deafness (2nd ed.)
by Peter V. Paul, Ph.D., and Stephen P. Quigley, Ph.D.

Study Guide for Language and Deafness (2nd ed.)
by Peter V. Paul, Ph.D.

Instructor's Manual for Language and Deafness (2nd ed.)
by Peter V. Paul, Ph.D.

Optimizing Theories and Experiments
by Randall R. Robey, Ph.D., and Martin C. Schultz, Ph.D.

Neuroscience of Communication
by Douglas B. Webster, Ph.D.

Professional Issues in Communication Disorders
edited by Rosemary Lubinski, Ed.D., and Carol Frattali, Ph.D.

Also available
A Singular Manual of Textbook Preparation by M. N. Hegde, Ph.D.

NEUROSCIENCE OF COMMUNICATION

Douglas B. Webster, Ph.D.

Louisiana State University Medical Center
New Orleans, Louisiana

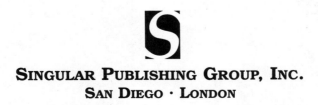

SINGULAR PUBLISHING GROUP, INC.
SAN DIEGO · LONDON

Singular Publishing Group, Inc.
4284 41st Street
San Diego, California 92105-1197

19 Compton Terrace
London, N1 2UN, UK

©1995 by Singular Publishing Group, Inc.

Typeset in 10½/12½ Bookman by So Cal Graphics
Printed in the United States of America by BookCrafters

Library of Congress Cataloging-in-Publication Data

Webster, Douglas B., 1934–
   Neuroscience of communication / Douglas B. Webster.
      p.   cm.
   Includes bibliographical references and index.
   ISBN 1-56593-114-9
   1. Communication disorders—Physiological aspects.   2. Brain—Diseases.
3. Neurolinguistics.   4. Neurobiology.   I. Title.
RC423.W312 1995
616.85'507—dc20   95–15661
                                             CIP

CONTENTS

Section II   Balance and Hearing

Section III   Speech and Language

PREFACE

The ultimate control of speech, hearing, and language lies in the brain. It follows, therefore, that in order to keep up with their field and serve their clients, today's communication sciences professionals need a comprehensive understanding of neuroscience. Such knowledge also forms the basis for interpreting once-exotic objective tests of communication abilities—such as evoked potentials, magnetic resonance imaging, and otoacoustic emissions—which are rapidly becoming a part of the repertoire of the successful speech-language-hearing professional.

After teaching anatomy and physiology to communication sciences students for over 20 years, I became convinced of the need for a neuroscience textbook written specifically for this field. So I offer this contribution. It is intended to serve graduate and undergraduate students in a one-semester course and to act as a source for practicing clinicians whose formal training lacked depth in neuroscience. By design, it does not cover molecular biology, genetics, the specifics of neurotransmitters, or other important but tangential fields.

The book assumes no background in biology, chemistry, or physics. It does assume a lively intellectual curiosity about the brain and how it works, and it endeavors to nurture that curiosity into a deepened understanding.

All chapters and their major subdivisions have summaries; each chapter has a "study guide" of pertinent questions to help the student review. There are marginal notes and boxes throughout that contain additional information or perspectives. Important terms are printed in bold faced type and indexed; the index entries guide the student to the definitions. There are a few suggestions for additional readings at the end of each chapter; each of the cited works is a standard in the field and each contains extensive references to more detailed literature.

The 10 chapters are organized into three sections.

Section I, Fundamentals, provides basic information about the brain's structural and functional organization. Chapter 1 introduces the brain's structure and function and provides an historical summary of the development of major concepts in neuroscience. Chapter 2 explains the functional anatomy of nerve cells and the relationships of nerves and muscles. Chapter 3 describes the surface anatomy of the brain and its blood supply. Chapter 4 explores the brain's internal organization.

Sections II, Balance and Hearing, and III, Speech and Language, delve in detail into the aspects of neuroscience that are of primary concern to the communication scientist and clinician. In Section II, Chapter 5 presents the vestibular system and Chapters 6 and 7, the peripheral and central auditory systems. In Section III, Chapter 8 discusses cerebral cortical organization and speech reception and Chapter 9, the neurobiology of language organization. Finally, Chapter 10 describes the complex and fascinating subject of speech production.

The illustrations were prepared by Gina Laurent and my wife, Molly Webster, whose skill, artistry, and dedication to detail I greatly appreciate. I was fortunate once again to be able to take advantage of Molly Webster's professional writing and editing skills. The clarity and readability of the text reflect her considerable talents.

Finally, I thank the good folks at Singular Publishing Group—particularly Marie Linvill and Sandy Doyle—for their support and encouragement throughout the gestation and preparation of this book.

A student once said, "You make a boring subject fascinating." Although I appreciated the compliment, I hold a different view: there is nothing *more* fascinating than neuroscience, if properly understood. It underlies every part of our humanity and makes us who and what we are. And our abilities to communicate with and understand others of our species are major defining aspects of our humanity. I hope that this book will help professionals in the communication sciences not only to understand but to appreciate the beauty and wonder of those abilities.

SECTION I

Fundamentals

In order to understand the neuroscience of communication, you must first understand the basic anatomy and physiology of the entire nervous system. Without this perspective, you would have no context for the details of balance, hearing, speech, and language.

This four chapter section gives you such a perspective by introducing you to

- the field of neuroscience (Chapter 1),
- the cellular organization of the nervous system (Chapter 2),
- the overall organization of the nervous system (Chapter 3), and
- the internal structure of the central nervous system (Chapter 4).

1

INTRODUCTION AND HISTORICAL PERSPECTIVES

The human brain is the supreme organ of the body. Within the brain we perceive, think, know, fear, love, hate, make decisions, and initiate and control our actions. The brain defines who we are.

The intellectual discipline that studies the brain is Neuroscience, a branch of science that did not even exist until the mid-1960s. Prior to that, anatomy, physiology, embryology, psychology, psychiatry, pharmacology, biochemistry, neurology, and neurosurgery all looked at the brain but, with rare exceptions, saw it piecemeal. There was little communication between these fields, and an expert in one was often not knowledgeable in another.

Since the mid-1960s, however, brain studies in these separate fields have been gradually merged into Neuroscience. During the same period there have been astounding advances in the tools and techniques for studying the brain. As a result, we have a much more cohesive understanding of this organ today than we did a generation ago.

I. NEUROSCIENCE AND COMMUNICATION DISORDERS

The field of Neuroscience is of particular importance to speech, hearing, and language professionals. Speech production requires intricate, precise control of many muscles: in the thorax (chest); in the neck, particularly the pharynx and larynx; and in the head (jaw, tongue, palate, and face). Speech, like any other muscular activity, is controlled by the brain through nerves that activate muscles, causing each to contract at just the right time and to just the right extent. To understand either normal or abnormal speech, we must understand brain mechanisms.

The brain is also paramount in hearing. The ear detects the vibrations of sound, changes them to nerve impulses, and sends them to the brain, but it is the brain that decodes and interprets them. To understand hearing, normal or abnormal, we must understand the neuromechanisms by which a code of neural impulses is changed into a perception of meaningful sounds.

Then there is language—totally an activity of the brain, in which ideas are formulated following internalized logic or rules (e.g., of English, French, American Sign Language, symbolic logic, or some other language). The words or signs of the language are the symbols that give shape to our thoughts. They are also the means of expressing our thoughts if, after formulating the idea, we send the language to the motor part of the brain and it becomes manifest. Therefore, as with speech and hearing, understanding brain mechanisms is essential to understanding language.

The goal of this textbook is to help you do just that—understand the mechanisms of the brain and peripheral nervous system that underlie the wondrously flexible systems of speech, language, and hearing.

A. Organization of the Nervous System

The nervous system is divided into central and peripheral parts. The **central nervous system (CNS)** consists of the brain, which lies within the cranial cavity of the skull, and the spinal cord, which lies within a bony canal of the vertebral column. The **peripheral nervous system (PNS)** consists of peripheral nerves that go between the central nervous system and other parts of the body.

All parts of the body are composed of fundamental building blocks called cells or of the products of cells (extracellular material) (Figure 1–1). In the nervous system there are two types of cells: **neurons** (nerve cells), which transmit information, usually in the form of nerve impulses, and **satellite cells**, which in various ways facilitate neurons but do not transmit nerve impulses.

Surprisingly, there are many more satellite cells than neurons in the nervous system.

The primary function of the nervous system is communication. Neurons have developed many specializations for communication characteristics that set them apart from other cells and that facilitate rapid propagation of nerve impulses and transmission of messages from one cell to another.

B. Neurons and Their Arrangements

Like other cells of the body, neurons contain a nucleus and various other organelles necessary for the cell's functioning. Most organelles are contained in the portion of the cell called the **cell body**, or **soma**. Unlike most other cells, neurons have processes that extend variable distances from the cell body. Most neurons have two types of processes: a group of shorter processes called **dendrites**, and a single,

There are more details about neurons and their organelles in Chapter 2.

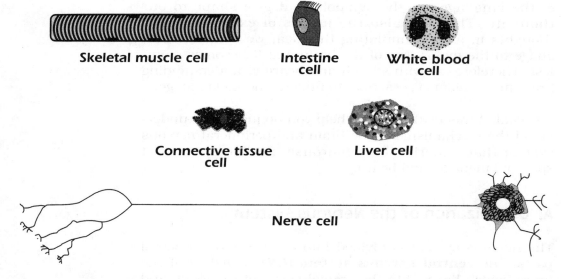

Figure 1–1. Nerve cells differ from other cells of the body in several ways including having long processes and the ability to propagate nerve impulses.

longer process called the **axon** (Figure 1–1). Although the axon is often less than a millimeter in length (see the following box, "Measurements"), in the largest neurons it can be as long as a meter. For instance, some axons from neurons whose cell bodies are in your brain extend to the small of your back. Some axons of spinal cord neurons in the small of your back extend to your toes.

More about nerve impulses in Chapter 2.

Axons transmit messages in the form of nerve impulses. Nerve impulses are chemical-electrical signals that can travel from one part of the body to another at speeds up to a few hundred meters per second. Although that is less than the speed of electricity or light, it is rapid enough for efficient communication between distant parts of the body.

Neurons are not randomly scattered throughout the nervous system. Instead, their cell bodies are packed together in specific groups at discrete, identifiable locations.

A group of neuronal cell bodies and their dendrites lying together is called a **ganglion** if it is in the peripheral nervous system, and a **nucleus** if it is in the central nervous system. When a group of neuronal cell bodies and their dendrites form a flat sheet on the brain's surface, it is called a **cortex**.

Large numbers of neuronal fibers that course together are called **tracts** in the central nervous system, or **nerves** in

MEASUREMENTS

Like all sciences, Neuroscience uses the metric system of measurements. The metric system is a decimal system, using multiples of 10 (e.g., 10 millimeters in a centimeter) instead of multiples of 12 (e.g., 12 inches in a foot). Here are some equivalents:

1 meter (m)		39.37 inches
1 centimeter (cm)	(1/100th of a meter)	00.39 inches
1 millimeter (mm)	1/1000th of a meter)	00.039 inches
1 micrometer (μm)	1/1,000,000 of a meter)	00.000039 inches
1 liter (l)		61.025 cubic inches
1 milliliter (ml)	1/1000th of a liter	00.061 cubic inches
1 gram (g)		00.0022 pounds
1 kilogram (kg)	(1000 grams)	02.2 pounds

the peripheral nervous system. They are referred to collectively as the **white matter**, because in fresh specimens many of them have a glistening white fatty covering called the **myelin sheath**. Cell bodies lack this myelin sheath and appear gray in fresh specimens; therefore ganglia, nuclei, or cortices collectively are called **gray matter**.

Information passes from one neuron to another at the **synapse**, an area where the endings of one neuron's processes are closely approximated to some portion of another neuron. When a nerve impulse comes to the end of an axon, it causes a chemical, called a **neurotransmitter**, to be released at the synapse. This neurotransmitter either excites or inhibits the next neuron; that is, it either facilitates the next neuron to start sending nerve impulses, or inhibits it from doing so (Figure 1–2). Thus the information passed from one neuron to another is either excitatory or inhibitory, depending on its effect on the next neuron.

Details of synaptic anatomy and physiology are in Chapter 2.

C. Three Functional Types of Neurons

Neurons that cause muscles to contract or glands to secrete are called **motor neurons** because their excitation causes movement, which is motor activity. Many motor neurons send nerve impulses out of the brain or spinal cord through their axons, which are the motor fibers of the peripheral nerves (Figure 1–3). Because they carry information away from the central nervous system, they are also called **efferent neurons**.

Neurons are also classified by the number of processes they have. Chapter 2 explains this.

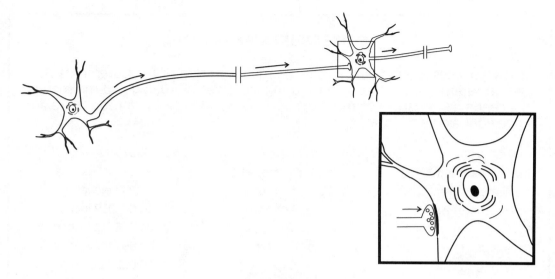

Figure 1–2. Nerve cells communicate with other nerve cells via neurotransmitters at synapses. This diagram shows a nerve impulse going to a nerve ending that then releases neurotransmitters to another neuron at a synapse. If the neurotransmitters excite the nerve cell sufficiently, nerve impulses are propagated down the second neuron's axon.

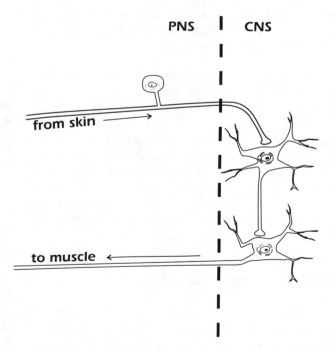

PNS | CNS

from skin →

to muscle ←

Figure 1–3. Diagram of the neuronal circuitry of a simple reflex. Sensory neurons from the skin propagate nerve impulses to the CNS and synapse with small interneurons whose axons synapse with motor neurons whose axons leave the CNS to synapse on muscle cells. In this way, stimulation of the skin can result in muscular contractions.

Other neurons carry sensory information from the periphery into the central nervous system (Figure 1–3). They are thus called **sensory neurons**, or, because they carry information toward the central nervous system, **afferent neurons**.

There is another class of neurons, called **interneurons** or **internuncial neurons**. They lie within the central nervous system and process information carried by both sensory and motor neurons. The vast majority of neurons of the central nervous system are interneurons.

Summary

The nervous system is divided into the central nervous system (CNS) and the peripheral nervous system (PNS). Each is composed of nerve cells (neurons), which transmit nerve impulses, and satellite cells, which facilitate neurons. Information is transmitted from one neuron to another at a synapse, where a process of one neuron closely approximates another neuron. We classify neurons by their functions. There are motor neurons, sensory neurons, and interneurons.

II. BRAIN ORGANIZATION

Imagine proceeding upward from the spinal cord into the skull to examine the organization of the brain. The first part is the **medulla** (or **medulla oblongata**); it lies at the base of the skull and is directly continuous with the spinal cord. Above the medulla is the **pons** and above that, the **midbrain**. Together, the medulla, pons, and midbrain make up the **brainstem**. Attached to the posterior surface of the pons is the **cerebellum**, a large structure that lies in the back part of the cranial cavity of the skull.

Above the brainstem is the **diencephalon**, which means "between brain"—so-named because it lies between the brainstem and the **cerebral hemispheres** above and around it. The diencephalon and the cerebral hemispheres make up the forebrain.

These large divisions of the brain are further described in Chapter 3.

The right and left cerebral hemispheres form the **cerebrum**, which is by far the largest portion of the brain. The cerebral

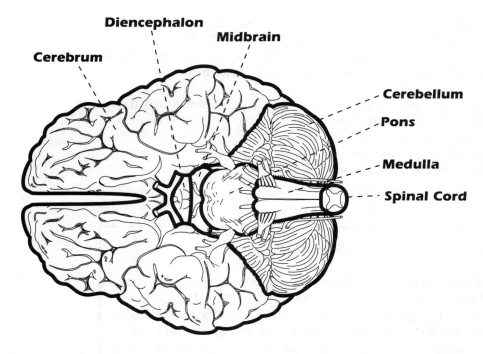

Figure 1–4. Diagram of the inferior surface of the brain showing the continuation of the spinal cord with the brain and the six major divisions of the brain.

hemispheres are entirely covered by sheets of gray matter, called **cerebral cortex**. Deep within, the cerebral hemispheres contain a great deal of both gray and white matter.

These portions of the brain—medulla, pons, midbrain, cerebellum, diencephalon, and cerebrum—are continuous with the spinal cord and with one another (Figure 1–4). They are not separate entities or discrete structures. Their boundaries, which are somewhat arbitrary, present no impediment to the flow of information.

A. Descriptors for the Brain

1. Terminology

One of the most difficult aspects of learning neuroscience is the large number of descriptive terms. There are many new words; and there are familiar words used in specialized ways. Moreover, some words mean one thing in one context and something different in another. Here are the most important descriptors used in human anatomy.

a. Terms of Direction **Anterior** means in front of—
that is, toward the front of the body. Conversely, **posterior**
means behind, or toward the back of the body. These are
terms that need a point of reference: for instance, the toes
are anterior to the heel.

Ventral is similar to anterior, except that it refers to what
was anterior during early development when the neural
tube, including the brain, was straight. During development
the neural tube bends almost 90° at the juncture of the
brainstem and diencephalon. Therefore, while ventral and
anterior refer to the same surface in the spinal cord and
brainstem, the ventral surfaces of the diencephalon and
cerebrum are their inferior surfaces (see below).

Dorsal is the converse of ventral. Therefore the dorsal surface of the cerebrum is its superior surface; the dorsal surface of the spinal cord is its posterior surface (see below).

Superior and **inferior** in human anatomical terminology
denote relative position only, not a value judgment. Superior means toward the top of the head; inferior means
toward the bottom of the feet. Thus, the spinal cord is inferior to the brain (Figure 1–5).

The terms **rostral** and **caudal** are only slightly different
than superior and inferior. Rostral means toward the head
(rostrum is Latin for beak); caudal means toward the tail
(caudal is Latin for tail). When they refer to structures in
the head, rostral means toward the nose (beak) and caudal
means toward the back of the head.

Proximal and **distal** describe the relative positions of parts
of a structure. Proximal means nearer the point where the
structure connects with the rest of the body. Conversely,
distal means farther from that point. Thus your elbow is
proximal to your wrist but distal to your shoulder. Proximal
and distal can also be used to describe smaller body parts.
For instance, the proximal part of an axon is near the cell
body; the distal part is near the terminal boutons.

Medial and **lateral** refer to positions relative to the midline
of the body. Medial means closer to the midline; lateral
means farther from the midline. Note that medial and middle are not synonymous: middle, as in everyday speech,
means between two things, or in the center of something.

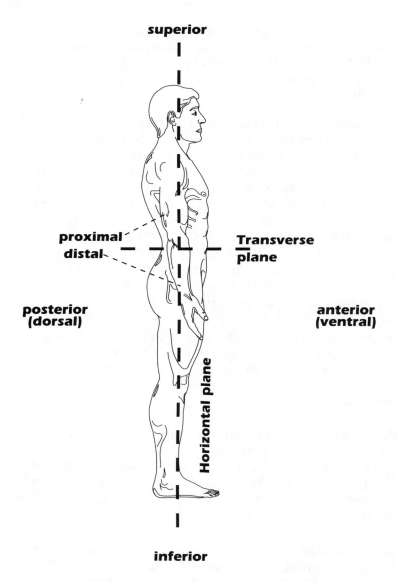

superior

proximal
distal

Transverse
plane

posterior
(dorsal)

anterior
(ventral)

Horizontal plane

inferior

Figure 1–5. Diagram showing some anatomic descriptors and planes.

Afferent and **efferent** are relative terms describing function. Afferent means to carry toward; efferent means to carry away from. Both terms need a point of reference. When the reference is to the cerebral cortex, afferent axons carry information to, and efferent axons carry information away from, the cerebral cortex. When the point of reference is not given, it is assumed to be either the CNS or the cerebral cortex. Thus an afferent system is a sensory system carrying information from the periphery to the CNS and usually, within the CNS, to the cerebral cortex.

b. Sections and Planes A cut through the body, or part of it, is called a section; the resulting cut surface is called a plane. A precise set of terminology describes sections and planes.

A **sagittal** section divides the body (or a midline organ of the body, such as the brain) into precise right-left halves, producing two equal, mirror-image pieces. A parasagittal section is parallel to the sagittal plane but not in the midline.

A **coronal** or **transverse** section of the CNS is at a right angle to the neuraxis. It is commonly called a cross-section. A coronal or transverse section of the spinal cord or brainstem is in the horizontal plane (parallel to the floor if the subject were standing upright). However, a coronal or transverse section of the diencephalon or cerebrum is in a vertical plane (at a right angle to the floor if the subject were standing upright).

A **horizontal** section is parallel to the neuraxis and at right angles to the sagittal plane.

B. Integration in the Nervous System

The parts of the nervous system function together to produce perception, thought, and action. As an example, let's consider what happens if you burn your finger on a hot stove, pull your hand away, and then pop your finger into your mouth.

The heat stimulates the skin of your finger and causes a series of nerve impulses that travel through peripheral sensory nerves in your finger, hand, wrist, and arm. The cell bodies of these sensory nerves lie in a ganglion just outside the spinal cord; their central fibers travel into the spinal cord and synapse on two other groups of neurons.

First there are interneurons, which lie completely within the spinal cord and synapse with motor neurons. The motor neurons extend out to muscles in your arm, which they excite; the muscles contract and your arm pulls your hand away from the hot stove. This is a **reflexive action**: all of the neural activity has occurred within the spinal cord and the peripheral nervous system of your arm. Because this activity does not involve the brain, it occurs very rapidly, before you are even consciously aware of the pain. Such

Some reflexes, such as the stapedius reflex, involve parts of the brain; however, all reflexes are nonvolitional.

rapid reflexes, which help you avoid injury, are highly adaptive to survival.

Except for olfaction, all information reaching the cerebral hemispheres is first processed in the diencephalon.

The sensory neurons also synapse with a second group of neurons, whose axons carry the pain information through the spinal cord and the entire brainstem and finally synapse on neurons in a particular nucleus of the diencephalon. These diencephalic neurons in turn send their axons up to the cerebral cortex, where you finally perceive the pain.

This is a longer route with more synapses than the reflexive route, which produced the immediate protective action, and it takes longer for nerve impulses to travel it. In other words, you pulled your hand away before you knew you were hurt. But now that you are consciously aware of the pain, hundreds of millions of neurons within your cerebral cortex go to work, comparing this experience with past experiences and deciding what to do about it.

As you will learn in Chapter 3, the cerebral cortex has four large lobes: the frontal, parietal, occipital, and temporal lobes.

The decision to put the injured finger into your mouth is made in the frontal portion of the cerebral cortex, called the **frontal lobe**. Once made, the decision requires a motor plan to activate the correct muscles in a precise temporal sequence. Therefore, the decision is sent from the frontal lobe to motor parts of the brain where the activity will be planned. These motor parts include still another portion of the cerebral cortex, portions of the deeper part of the cerebral hemisphere, and portions of the cerebellum. Nerve impulses travel from the cerebrum to motor neurons of the spinal cord, which send their axons to your arm muscles and cause them to contract. Finally the finger reaches the soothing environment of your mouth (Figure 1–6).

This is a simplified, although accurate, description of how a sensory stimulation (pain to your finger) can cause a reflex reaction (withdrawal), followed by conscious awareness and deliberate action. The information is carried through discrete neural pathways (groups of axons running together, called tracts) to the cerebral cortex where pain is perceived and decisions made. By the end of this textbook you will understand more of the associated bells and whistles. The important point for now, and a major emphasis of this book, is that there are biological explanations for how our nervous system receives, processes, and acts on information. Clinicians must understand these normal neural pathways and functions in order to deal appropriately with abnormal events, including those affecting speech, language, and hearing.

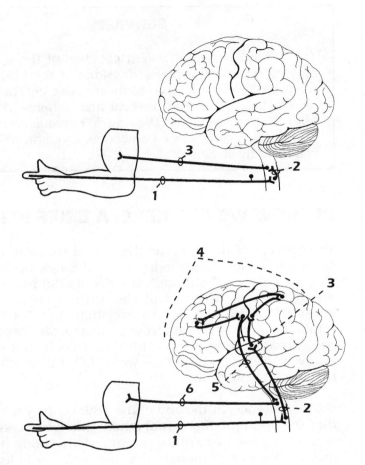

Figure 1–6. Diagram of the neural and muscular events that result when you burn a finger. There are both reflexive and cerebral circuits. In the reflex *(upper picture),* a sensory nerve (1) brings the information to the spinal cord and synapses with an interneuron (2) in the spinal cord; the interneuron then synapses with a motor neuron (3) that goes to your arm muscles, which withdraw the finger from the heat. In the cerebral involvement *(lower picture),* a sensory nerve (1) brings the information to the spinal cord and synapses with neurons (2) that carry the information to the diencephalon deep in the brain (3); the diencephalon relays the pain information to the cerebral cortex (4) where you consider the situation and decide what to do. After you decide to put your finger in your mouth, the cerebral cortex sends this information to the spinal cord (5) where there are synapses with motor neurons that innervate muscles of your arm and hand; these neurons send the command "put finger in mouth" to the appropriate muscles (6).

Summary

The central nervous system consists of the spinal cord and the brain. The major divisions of the brain are the medulla, the pons, the midbrain, the cerebellum, the diencephalon, and the cerebral hemispheres. All parts of both the peripheral and the central nervous systems function together to produce perception, thought, reflexes, and volitional movements.

III. HOW WE GOT HERE: A BRIEF HISTORY

The concept of the brain as the seat of thought, comprehension, perception, and bodily control dates back to ancient Greek civilization, although the details did not emerge until much later. By the end of the 18th century, the brain's gross anatomy had been described, but its functioning remained a mystery. Inferences based on dissections and behavioral observations—which had been profitable in the study of other body parts—were difficult or impossible in the study of the brain.

So, for instance, at the end of the 18th century it was thought that the brain produced vital ethers that were passed through hollow nerves to various organs of the body and caused motion. It was also thought that the brain, or at least its cerebral hemispheres, acted as a whole and that different parts did not have specific different functions.

A. Localization of Function

During the 19th century, clinical observations on humans, combined with electrical stimulation of the cortex in experimental animals, led to two opposing views: (1) that there is a great deal of functional localization in the cerebral hemispheres and (2) that the cerebral hemispheres act as a holistic unit rather than as several parts. Although neither of these extremes proved correct, it was gradually established that there is indeed a great deal of localization of function in the brain.

The first dramatic example was **Paul Broca's** demonstration that destruction of a discrete portion of the human left inferior frontal cortex damaged speech production but caused no loss of language comprehension or of motor abilities, even in the larynx. This suggested that the left inferior frontal cortex quite specifically controls expressive speech.

Other clinical observations supported the concept of functional localization. **Karl Wernicke**, for example, found that damage in the posterior part of the left superior temporal cortex resulted in a loss of speech comprehension.

Equally noteworthy were observations on persons with epilepsy, made in England by **Hulings Jackson**. He saw that an epileptic seizure started in one small area of the body and then radiated systematically to adjoining parts of the body. Postmortem examination of the brains of these persons always showed an area of the cerebral cortex with damaged neurons. Jackson assumed that the seizure started with these damaged neurons and that these cortical areas were correlated with the body areas where the seizure first manifested itself. He concluded that there is a strip of cortex in the posterior part of the frontal lobe that represents motor activity and that different parts of the opposite side of the body are represented in specific parts of this strip.

At the same time, other scientists were finding that electrical stimulation of specific parts of the cerebral cortex of experimental animals caused movements of specific muscle groups. These observations confirmed Jackson's conclusions.

Such observations and experiments further bolstered the idea that specific brain functions are localized in specific areas of the cortex. It was widely believed in the late 19th century that each portion of the cerebral cortex was responsible for a specific function or quality, with one portion for love, another for hate, a third for sexual drive, and so on. It was further thought that, if a person had one of these qualities in excess, the relevant portion of the cerebrum would grow larger than normal and would create a corresponding bump on the skull above it. Thus was born the pseudo-science of **phrenology**, which became quite popular in the late 19th and early 20th centuries. It purported to be able to describe—even to predict—personality and behavior based on the configuration of a person's skull.

However, no correlation between bumps on the head and personality or abilities was found, and the idea of such extreme localization of function was eventually discredited. The pendulum swung back to the idea that the cerebrum acts as a whole, rather than as separate, independent parts.

It is interesting that we still tend to judge people's personalities and abilities by their looks.

Various experiments explored this idea, most notably those by **Carl Lashley** during the first third of the 20th century. Lashley worked with rats that had learned to run a complex maze. He could find no single cerebral area whose destruction would also destroy the ability to run the maze. However, he did find that the more cortex he removed, the greater the total deficit in maze-running behavior became. The discovery that the extent of brain damage was more important than its location seemed to reinforce the older idea that the cortex acted as a unit.

Today, from our perspective at least, the pendulum has centered. We now understand that discrete functions are indeed localized within specific areas of the cerebral cortex. We also know that higher order functions, such as attention and thought, involve large areas of the cortex as well as other parts of the brain. We will deal with these phenomena in later portions of this book.

B. The Cell Theory

During the 19th and 20th centuries there have been many other advances in our understanding of the brain—and, indeed, of all biology. In the 1830s there was a major intellectual breakthrough when **Matthias Schleiden** and **Theodor Schwann** first enunciated the **Cell Theory**. This theory, made possible by the invention of the compound microscope, states that all parts of the body are made up of cells or products of cells. Enthusiastic, hard-working early microscopists demonstrated this to be true in all tissues except the nervous system.

Nervous tissue just did not look the same to them, however, and for good reason: it was those processes, traveling together in tracts and unique to the nervous system. Although the nucleus-containing cell bodies of neurons were familiar and easy to identify, the tracts were mystifying. The early microscopists were not certain that they were parts of cells, and many concluded that the nervous system was the exception to the Cell Theory.

C. The Neuron Doctrine

By the latter half of the 19th century, new techniques of study were available. Of particular note is the Golgi method, developed by **Camillo Golgi** in 1873 and still in use today, which stains an entire neuron—cell body, axon, and dendrites. At last it was possible to see the extent of an individual neuron.

But the new method introduced another new theory. Golgi himself, carefully describing the cells and processes in his preparations, thought he saw fine continuities between the processes of different nerve cells. However, this contradicted the Cell Theory, which declared that there were no continuities between cells. If Golgi's observations were correct, it would mean that each nerve "cell" was not a separate entity. He proposed instead a **"Reticular Theory"** of the nervous system. It stated that there was continuity between the different elements of the nervous system, which he understood to be a large composite rather than separate cells.

On the other side of this discussion was a Spanish neuroanatomist, **Santiago Ramón y Cajal**, who not only used Golgi's techniques with precision and elegance but also improved on them. The conclusion he drew from his preparations was that processes from one neuron came close to those of another, and even intermingled, but did not interconnect. There was, he said, no continuity of protoplasm between neurons.

Golgi and Cajal shared a Nobel Prize in Physiology and Medicine in 1906.

As more investigators examined the question, Cajal's view came to prevail. Since the 1950s, electron microscopy has confirmed that indeed there is no continuity between neurons. Cajal is credited with formulating the **Neuron Doctrine**—that each neuron is a separate cell—even though it was not he but another great European anatomist, **Wilhelm Waldeyer**, who first stated it in 1891.

D. Other Laws and Theories

At the same time the Cell Theory was being tested in the nervous system and the Neuron Doctrine was being developed, other attributes of the nervous system were being uncovered.

For instance, investigators were coming to understand the functional difference between motor neurons, which carry information out to the periphery, and sensory neurons, which carry information into the central nervous system.

Others were realizing that peripheral nerves to and from the spinal cord segregate their sensory and motor neurons: sensory neurons enter the cord dorsally, through the "dorsal nerve root;" motor neurons leave the cord ventrally, through the "ventral nerve root;" then the sensory and motor components fuse to form the peripheral nerve. This principle—that the dorsal nerve root is only sensory and the ventral nerve root only motor—is named the **Bell-Magendie Law** for **Sir Charles Bell** and **François Magendie**, who first stated it.

E. Law of Specific Nerve Energies

Johannes Müller of Germany enunciated the **Law of Specific Nerve Energies** in 1833. It states that when a nerve is stimulated, the information it carries is determined not by the stimulus but by where its fibers terminate. For example, when light stimulates the eye, the nerve impulses it sets up are carried by the optic nerve to the brain where the stimulus is perceived as light. However, a blow to the eye or head can also stimulate nerve impulses in these fibers, and these will also be perceived as light: the well-known and painful phenomenon of "seeing stars."

F. Specificity of Neural Connections

We are still learning just how axons find— or seek out— their appropriate destinations.

The Law of Specific Nerve Energies helped explain the localization of function within the brain. Cajal carried it a step further with a proposition about the specificity of neural connections. This proposition states that, as a neuron develops, its axon seeks out certain structures, or targets, within the brain and makes connections with them. In other words, axons do not wander about making random terminations, even during development; each nerve or group of nerves has specific, predetermined destinations and contacts.

G. Dynamic Polarization of Neurons

Cajal presented a second Law: **On the Dynamic Polarization of Neurons**. It states that neurons transmit information in only one direction: dendrites transmit toward the cell body; axons transmit away from the cell body; neither ever transmits in the opposite direction. Although there are exceptions to this biological law, as there are with most biological laws, it has proven true as a generalization.

1. The Synapse

At the end of the 19th century another major concept was added to this developing picture: that of the synapse. The term was introduced by a British scientist, **Sir Charles Sherrington**, who was the first person to determine the neurophysiological bases for reflexes. He described how sensory information is brought into the central nervous system by sensory nerves that contact motor neurons via one or more interneurons and then send information out to muscles. In 1897, he had given the name **synapse** to the contacts between neurons where information is passed from one neuron to the next—and which we now know are not actual contacts but areas of close approximation.

Sherrington arrived at the concept of the synapse by a logical deduction that explained his physiological findings. He never saw a synapse, but had no doubt of its reality.

The synapse and Cajal's proposition of dynamic polarization provided pivotal pieces in the puzzle. It was now clear how neuronal pathways can carry specific information from one part of the nervous system to another.

Summary

By the end of the 18th century the gross anatomy of the brain was well described, but its functioning was only dimly understood. During the 19th century the Neuron Doctrine was proposed, the microscopic anatomy of the brain described, and much was learned about functional localization in the brain. The Law of Specific Nerve Energies and the realization of the specificity of neural connections, the dynamic polarization of neurons, and the concept of the synapse all paved the way toward an understanding of brain physiology.

IV. WHERE WE ARE TODAY

Thus, by the middle third of the 20th century, the nervous system was understood to be made up of dynamically polarized neurons, whose processes are arranged in groups and make specific neural connections by way of synapses. The way was prepared for the explosion of knowledge about nervous system organization and function that has been an intellectual hallmark of the decades that followed. What has been learned in these exciting years has dramatically changed many fields, including those of speech, hearing, and language.

CHAPTER 1 SUMMARY

The communication sciences of speech, language, and hearing are understandable only with a firm knowledge of neuroscience. The entire nervous system, peripheral and central, is composed of neurons and satellite cells. Sensory neurons transmit information from the periphery to various portions of the central nervous system. Motor neurons transmit information from the central nervous system to the effector organs—muscles and glands. Interneurons process information passing between sensory and motor systems.

The brain is subdivided into several parts: brainstem (medulla, pons, midbrain), cerebellum, diencephalon, and cerebral hemispheres. Sensory information from the periphery enters the central nervous system where it is processed and integrated. Motor activity (muscular contractions or glandular secretions) may be either nonvolitional reflexes or volitional movements, which are directed by the cerebral hemispheres.

Our survey of the nervous system began with what was known of its gross anatomy prior to the 19th century. Brain functioning and microscopic anatomy were studied extensively during the 19th century. Building on those 19th century discoveries and using new technologies, scientists of the 20th century have made great advances in understanding the structure, function, and biochemistry of the nervous system.

ADDITIONAL READING

Geschwind, N. (1963). Carl Wernicke, the Breslau school and the history of aphasia. In E. C. Carterette (Ed.), *Brain function, volume III: Speech, language, and communication* (pp. 1–16). Berkeley: University of California Press.

Shepherd, G. M. (1991). *Foundations of the neuron doctrine.* New York: Oxford University Press.

Sherrington, C. S. (1906). *The integrative action of the nervous system.* New Haven, CT: Yale University Press.

Taylor, G. R. (1963). *The science of life: A picture history of biology.* New York: McGraw-Hill.

Young, R. M. (1990) *Mind, brain, and adaptation in the nineteenth century.* New York: Oxford University Press.

STUDY GUIDE

Answer each question with a brief paragraph

1. What is neuroscience?

2. What structures make up the central nervous system?

3. What are the major parts of a neuron?

4. What is the difference between a nerve and a tract?

5. What is the functional difference between a sensory neuron and a motor neuron?

6. What is the brainstem?

7. Describe a reflex.

8. Give an example of localization of function in the brain.

9. Describe the Neuron Doctrine.

10. What is the Law of Specific Nerve Energies?

Odd One Out

In each of the following questions, choose the item that does not "fit" with the other three; briefly explain what the other three have in common that the odd one lacks. There may be more than one correct answer.

1. ____ soma
   ____ dendrite
   ____ satellite cell
   ____ axon
   WHY?

2. ___ ganglion
   ___ tract
   ___ nucleus
   ___ cortex
   WHY?

3. ___ midbrain
   ___ medulla
   ___ pons
   ___ cerebellum
   WHY?

4. ___ cerebrum
   ___ diencephalon
   ___ brainstem
   ___ spinal cord
   WHY?

5. ___ Neuron Doctorine
   ___ Reticular Theory
   ___ Cell Theory
   ___ Law of the Dynamic Polarization of Neurons
   WHY?

NERVE CELLS AND MUSCLES

How the nervous system works to control the rest of the body can be understood only if we first understand its component parts. In this chapter we will look at the parts of the nervous system and how they fit together—from the molecules that compose the cells to the organs that compose the system.

Cells have been called the building blocks of living organisms. Of course, as technology has allowed us to examine smaller and smaller entities, we have discovered that the building blocks themselves are composed of smaller units: cells contain tiny organs, called organelles; organelles are made up of molecules. At the opposite end of the scale, cells and their products make up all parts of both animals and plants and are organized into tissues, which are organized into organs, which are organized into systems.

I. GENERALIZED CELL STRUCTURE AND FUNCTION

A. Four Classes of Molecules

Living matter is composed of four major classes of organic molecules: **lipids, proteins, carbohydrates**, and **nucleic acids** (Table 2–1).

Table 2–1
Major organic molecules of cells.

Molecular Type	Component Parts	Common Name	Examples
Lipids	Fatty acids Glycerol	Fats Storage fats	Cell membranes
Proteins	Amino acids	Proteins	Enzymes Collagen
Carbohydrates	Simple sugars	Sugars	Table sugar Glycogen Starch
Nucleic acids	Nucleosides	Nucleic acids	Deoxyribonucleic acid (DNA) Ribonucleic acid (RNA)

1. Lipids

Lipids, commonly called fats, are composed of two smaller molecules—fatty acids and glycerol. Lipids are stored as body fat and seen as curves (or bulges), which are esthetically pleasing or not depending on fashion and point of view.

Lipids are a reserve energy supply for times when there is not enough food. They also contribute to essential structures: lipid molecules, arranged in two-layer sheets, form a vital part of the external covering of all cells and the outer layer of most organelles.

2. Proteins

Proteins are very large molecules. They are composed of smaller molecules called **amino acids** that are chemically bonded together into long strings, or chains. There are 21 common amino acids, not all of which are found in every protein. Some proteins contain only about 50 molecules of amino acids; others contain several hundred. Because the number, kind, and sequence of amino acid molecules in a protein determine its structural and functional characteristics, the potential number and variety of protein types is virtually limitless.

Some proteins are **structural proteins**: they are the major elements in structures such as muscle fibers, fingernails, tendons, and ligaments. Other proteins are **globular proteins**: they are usually either in solution or attached to lipid membranes. The most common globular proteins are **enzymes**—chemicals that facilitate and direct the body's chemical reactions.

3. Carbohydrates

Carbohydrates are commonly called sugars, although not all are sweet. They range from relatively small molecules, such as table sugar, to much larger molecules that are actually chains of small sugar molecules (much as proteins are chains of amino acids). These large sugar molecules are stored until they are needed. Then, with the help of the right enzymes, they are broken down into smaller sugar molecules and used in energy metabolism.

4. Nucleic Acids

Finally there are the nucleic acids: **deoxyribonucleic acid (DNA)** and **ribonucleic acid (RNA)**. These very large molecules provide the blueprints (the genetic code) for how cells are built, and the mechanisms for interpreting those blueprints.

B. Building a Cell

As you learn about cells and their parts, remember that they are microscopic in size. Even the largest and most complex cell can be seen only with a microscope.

As we have learned, the nervous system contains two types of cells: **neurons**, or nerve cells, which process information; and the more numerous **satellite cell**s, which facilitate the neurons' metabolism and functioning. Both types are specialized for their particular roles in the nervous system. They also share many characteristics of other cells. The following description of a generalized cell covers characteristics shared by almost all animal cells. The specializations that fit individual cells of the nervous system to their specific roles will be described in sections II and III of this chapter.

1. Bilipid Plasma Membrane

Each cell is totally enveloped by a **plasma membrane** which, because it includes a double layer of lipid molecules, is called a bilipid membrane. Each of the lipid molecules of the plasma membrane is chemically bonded to a protein molecule; together they form a complex molecule called a **lipoprotein**. The lipid portions of the lipoprotein molecules form the middle of the plasma membrane; the protein portions form the outer and inner layers of the plasma membrane (Figure 2–1). Because lipids do not dissolve in water, the lipids of the plasma membrane form a barrier between what is inside the cell (intracellular material) and what is outside (extracellular material).

2. Proteins in the Plasma Membrane

If the plasma membrane were composed entirely of lipoprotein molecules, however, most chemicals would not be able to get into or out of the cell; that is to say, there would be almost no communication between the cell's contents and the extracellular environment. That is not the case.

In fact, the bilipid membrane is studded with globular proteins (Figure 2–1). Some extend from the outside of the cell all the way through the membrane to the cell's contents; others are attached to either the outer or inner layer of the plasma membrane. When stimulated, these globular proteins allow certain dissolved molecules to pass through the

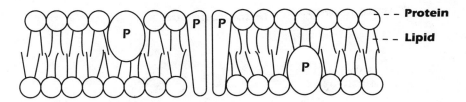

Figure 2–1. Schematic diagram of a plasma membrane showing the lipoprotein molecules (lipid plus protein) in two layers. Also shown, some large globular proteins (P), some of which act as channels for specific molecules.

plasma membrane; they are thus called "**channels**" in the membrane. Most channels are specific for just one type of molecule—that is, they allow only one type of dissolved molecule to pass through.

Ions—small molecules dissolved in extra- or intracellular fluid that carry either a positive or negative electric charge—are the most common molecules to pass through these channels.

Most channels open when a specific chemical is attached to the protein molecule from either inside or outside the cell. In this way, the cell responds to changes in its external or internal environment.

Some channel proteins are called "receptors" because specific extracellular molecules can attach to them (i.e., receive them) and thus activate (open or close) the channel.

3. Nucleus

The largest and most prominent organelle in a cell is its **nucleus** (Figure 2–2). Like the cell itself, the nucleus is bounded by a bilipid membrane. This nuclear membrane has several openings called pores.

The nucleus contains large concentrations of nucleic acids. Its DNA (deoxyribonucleic acid) is composed of very large molecules containing the blueprint (genetic code) for everything necessary to maintain the cell and to produce new cells. The nucleus also contains globular proteins; they attach to DNA molecules and regulate which portions of the genetic code are "active"—that is, can be "read" by RNA (ribonucleic acid) molecules at any given time.

The nucleus also contains a **nucleolus**. It is a small dense body, observable by light microscopy, that is formed of RNA

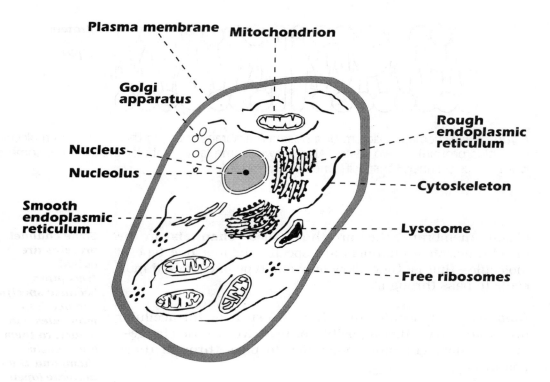

Figure 2–2. Schematic diagram of a generalized cell with its principle organelles.

and protein molecules. New RNA molecules are built in the nucleolus and transcribe the blueprint of the DNA; that is, they carry the information out of the nucleus and into the **cytosol** (the contents of a cell exclusive of the nucleus), where proteins are synthesized.

During cell division the DNA molecules line up and are held together by proteins; these are the **chromosomes**. At other times the DNA molecules are dispersed.

4. Mitochondria

Several organelles in the cytosol function for the livelihood (metabolism) of the cell. Most notable are the **mitochondria** (singular: mitochondrion). Mitochondria are bounded by a bilipid plasma membrane that is *not* derived from the cell's plasma membrane (Figure 2–2). In this respect it is unlike most other organelles of the cytosol.

Mitochondria have been called the "cell's powerhouses"; the more of them a cell has, the higher its metabolic rate. This is because enzymes in the mitochondria provide energy in the following manner:

- Oxygen and small sugar molecules are carried to cells by capillaries of the blood system. They enter the cell's cytosol through channels in the plasma membrane.
- The enzymes in the mitochondria, which require oxygen to act, use the oxygen thus supplied and break down the sugar molecules; that is, they break the chemical bonds that hold the atoms of the sugar together. Breaking the bonds releases energy and creates two waste products, carbon dioxide and water.
- The energy thus released is trapped by other molecules in the cell and used for cell metabolism. The carbon dioxide and water are resorbed into the bloodstream and eventually excreted from the body as waste products.
- If more small sugar molecules are brought to the cell than are needed for the cell's metabolism, the mitochondria synthesize them into a large sugar molecule called **glycogen**, which is stored as a reserve energy source for later use.

In addition to the enzymes that drive their energy production process, mitochondria also contain a small packet of DNA that gives instructions about making enzymes and other proteins.

5. Other Organelles (Infolded Membranes)

While mitochondria are bounded by their own distinct membranes, most other organelles in the cytosol are formed by infoldings of the cell's plasma membrane.

a. Smooth and Rough Endoplasmic Reticulum Sheets of bilipid membranes derived from the plasma membrane are found within the cytosol; they are called **smooth endoplasmic reticulum**.

In the electron microscope it can be seen that some endoplasmic reticulum is studded with small aggregates of RNA molecules, called **ribosomes**; it is called **rough endoplasmic reticulum**. Rough endoplasmic reticulum is formed by RNA molecules that have "read" the code for building new proteins from the nuclear DNA and then have moved out into the cytosol, through pores in the nuclear membrane, and attached to endoplasmic reticulum. The rough endo-plasmic reticulum therefore carries the precise code for building specific proteins. (Other ribosomes do not attach to endoplasmic reticulum but remain free in the cytosol.)

The building of new cellular proteins begins when an organism eats protein. For example, when you eat a piece of tender roast chicken your digestive system chemically breaks down large molecules of chicken protein into small amino acids. Your circulatory system carries them throughout your body; in the process, the amino acids diffuse out of the capillaries. They pass through channels into the cytosol of cells and are carried to the rough endoplasmic reticulum by ribosomes that have remained free in the cytosol. Energy produced by the mitochondria chemically links the amino acids in the appropriate order, as determined by the code carried by the RNA, and the specific human proteins your body cells need are formed.

b. Golgi Apparatus Most cells secrete proteins or large sugars. Secretion is accomplished by the **Golgi apparatus**—flattened bags of endoplasmic reticulum that lie in the cytosol. Protein or large sugar molecules become incorporated into the bags, or vesicles, which move to the cell's perimeter, fuse with it, and then secrete (extrude) their contents into the extracellular space.

For instance, digestive cells in the walls of the intestines produce enzymes that break down ingested proteins. The Golgi apparatus packages these enzymes and secretes them into the lumen (space) within the intestine. There the enzymes break the chemical bonds of large protein molecules—for instance, from the chicken in the example above. The amino acids that are freed when the bonds are broken are absorbed into the blood stream.

c. Lysosomes Smooth endoplasmic reticulum also forms **lysosomes**, which contain many enzymes and function as the cell's detoxifier and recycling plant. Used molecules are moved into the lysosomes and then broken up by the lysosomes' degrading enzymes; this destroys toxic products and allows the molecules to be recycled back into the cytosol where they are used for cell metabolism. If the used molecules cannot be recycled, they are extruded from the cell.

6. Cytoskeleton

Finally, each cell contains a kind of skeleton, called the **cytoskeleton**. This organelle is derived not from the plasma membrane, but from structural proteins. Some of these structural proteins are arranged in small filaments, called **microfilaments**; others form hollow **microtubules**. The cytoskeleton has two functions: it helps maintain the cell's shape; and it is an intracellular transport system that moves molecules from one part of the cell to another.

C. From Cells to Systems

As we have seen, each cell has many characteristics of an independent organism:

- an outer skin, the plasma membrane;
- shape-maintaining molecules, the cytoskeleton;
- DNA, which contains the plans for building all the materials necessary for life and reproduction.

It also has several of the functional abilities of an independent organism and, like an organism with specialized organs, carries on a myriad of functions. It can:

- store energy (in the mitochondria);
- build new large molecules (in the rough endoplasmic reticulum);
- move material out of the cell (by the Golgi apparatus);
- recycle used materials (by the lysosomes).

In a multicellular organism, the cells are only one of the levels of organization.

- Groups of cells working with one another to carry out similar functions are called **tissues** (e.g., nervous tissue, muscle tissue).
- A group of tissues functioning together is an **organ** (e.g., liver, kidney, stomach).
- A group of organs functioning together is an **organ system** (e.g., the liver, stomach, intestines, esophagus, etc. make up the digestive system).
- All the organ systems together comprise the **organism**.

We have now discovered a hierarchy of structures (Figure 2–3). It begins with the four types of organic molecules that make up

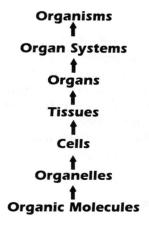

Figure 2–3. The hierarchy of structures that comprise an organism such as a person.

all living matter; continues through organelles to cells; and includes tissues, organs, organ systems, and organisms.

Summary

All living matter is composed of lipids, proteins, carbohydrates, and nucleic acids. In each cell, these molecules form organelles: plasma membrane, nucleus, mitochondria, endoplasmic reticulum (smooth and rough), Golgi apparatus, lysosomes, and cytoskeleton. Cells form tissues, which form organs, which form organ systems, which form organisms.

II. GENERAL STRUCTURE OF MULTIPOLAR NEURONS

The nervous system provides the rapid communication necessary to coordinate all levels of the hierarchy so that they can work together. Both neurons and satellite cells are specialized for their roles. The following discussion focuses on **multipolar neurons**, which are the most numerous type of neuron.

A. Processes

The most prominent specializations that distinguish neurons from other cells are their processes (Figure 2–4). There are two types, **axons** and **dendrites**; both are long, narrow extensions of cytosol from the main body of the cell. Processes greatly increase the cell's surface area (and plasma membrane) relative to its total mass. Their length puts some parts of the neuron at great distances (as much as 1 meter) from its metabolic center. In order to sustain these distant parts, neurons must have a high metabolic rate.

B. Nissl Substance

Neurons constantly produce many proteins, which are needed for membrane upkeep and information processing. The rough endoplasmic reticulum, which synthesizes proteins, is so prominent in neurons that it is given a special name, the **Nissl substance**.

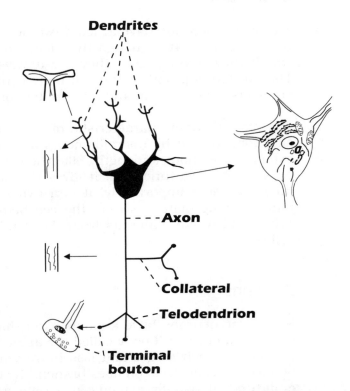

Figure 2–4. Outline of a multipolar neuron with details of its component parts.

C. Mitochondria

Unlike most cells, neurons do not store glycogen as a reserve energy supply; therefore they need a constant supply of oxygen and sugars. When there is insufficient oxygen—for instance, with a "blue baby" or a person suffering from asphyxia—brain cells are the first to die; and they cannot be replaced. To meet this need, neurons have more mitochondria than most other cells.

D. Cell Body

"Perikaryon" means the region around (peri-) the nucleus of the cell.

In all cells, the major organelles—Nissl substance, mitochondria, smooth endoplasmic reticulum, Golgi apparatus, and lysosomes—are concentrated in the area of the cell immediately surrounding the nucleus. In neurons, the processes extend from this same part of the cell, called the neuronal **cell body**, or **soma**, or **perikaryon**.

E. Dendrites

Multipolar neurons have at least two dendrites and usually more (Figure 2–4). Although their lengths and the extent to which they branch vary, they are always relatively short. The portion adjacent to the cell body contains some rough endoplasmic reticulum and a few mitochondria.

The most distinct characteristic of the dendrite is its cytoskeleton, formed by microfilaments and microtubules that extend throughout its length. Like the cytoskeleton of other cells, it has two functions. It gives the dendrite structural integrity. More importantly, it is a two-way transport system, carrying materials from the cell body out to the dendrites and waste materials from the dendrites back to the cell body.

F. Axons

Multipolar neurons have a single axon that extends from a small area of the cell body called the **axon hillock**. The axon is usually much longer and less branched than any of the dendrites. When an axon does branch, the branch is called a **collateral**; it usually extends at a right angle to the axon, rather than at an acute angle as do dendritic branches.

Both the axon and the axon hillock contain very few organelles. However, the axon has an extremely well organized cytoskeleton that, as in dendrites, functions for both structural integrity and the transport of chemicals between the cell body and distant parts of the axon. Although this transport system is essentially the same as that in dendrites, for historical reasons it is called **axoplasmic transport** in axons. It is necessary for the axon's livelihood.

G. Terminal Bouton

At the end of each axon and collateral there is a swelling called a **terminal bouton** (Figure 2–4). Just before the terminal bouton there are usually short axonal branches, called **telodendria**, each of which has its own terminal bouton.

"Telodendria" is plural. The singular is "telodendrion."

The terminal bouton contains mitochondria, which as usual provide energy, and a cytoskeleton. But the most characteristic feature of the terminal bouton is a large number of tiny, smooth, hollow spheres of membranes—the **synaptic vesicles**. They are usually clustered together in the part of the terminal bouton that is adjacent to a portion of another neuron's plasma membrane. The space between the terminal bouton and the plasma membrane of the next neuron is the **synaptic cleft**. The terminal bouton and adjacent plasma membrane of the other neuron together form the **synapse**; the portion of the adjacent neuron's plasma membrane is the **postsynaptic membrane** (Figure 2–5).

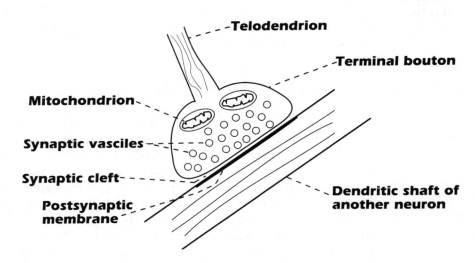

Figure 2–5. Diagram of a terminal bouton and postsynaptic membrane forming a synapse.

Summary

Most CNS neurons are multipolar. They have two or more dendrites and a single axon. All processes emanate from the cell body, which contains Nissl substance and numerous mitochondria. Axonal endings, named terminal boutons, contain synaptic vesicles. The terminal bouton and the plasma membrane of the adjacent neuron comprise the synapse.

III. SPECIAL PHYSIOLOGY OF NERVE CELLS

All cells have the general characteristic of "**irritability**." Without it, they would not have physiological responses to outside influences. This characteristic is particularly well developed in neurons.

A. Resting Potentials

A millivolt, abbreviated mV, is 1/1,000 of a volt; the standard flashlight battery carries 1.5 volts.

One aspect of irritability (shared by all cells) is the **resting potential**. Simply stated, this means that the cell's cytosol is electrically negative relative to the extracellular fluid, usually by about 70 millivolts (mV). As electrical potentials go, the resting potential's 70/1000 of a volt is not much; but at the level of cellular activity it is substantial. The resting potential is maintained by the balance of negative to positive ions, that is, there are more negative and fewer positive ions inside the cell, and more positive and fewer negative ions outside the cell.

B. Graded (Local) Potentials

When a mechanical or chemical event affects a neuron's plasma membrane, it is called a "**perturbation**"; the neuron is said to be "perturbed." Perturbations may either excite or inhibit a cell. When a perturbation is excitatory, the plasma membrane channels open, which causes negative ions to flow out and/or positive ions to flow in. The resting potential becomes less than -70 mV in that portion of the cell. This is a **depolarization**, called an excitatory **local (graded) potential**. It can occur in the soma or along a dendrite, or, in some cases, on the initial portion of an axon.

Some kinds of chemicals perturb the cell membrane in such a way that the ion channels that are opened cause negative ions to flow in, or positive ions to flow out, or both. This reversal of the excitatory pattern increases the negativity inside the cell, making the resting potential greater than − 70 mV; this is not depolarization, but rather **hyperpolarization**, and is called an inhibitory local (graded) potential.

Once started, graded potentials spread down dendrites or through the cell body to other parts of the cell. However, as they extend further away from the site of perturbation, they become smaller, that is, they **decrement**. By the time a graded potential that began with a perturbation at the end of a dendrite reaches the cell body, the change in potential may be negligible (Figure 2–6).

C. Action Potentials: Nerve Impulses

When there is a depolarization of about 15 mV (depending on the neuron) at the axon hillock, it causes an **action**

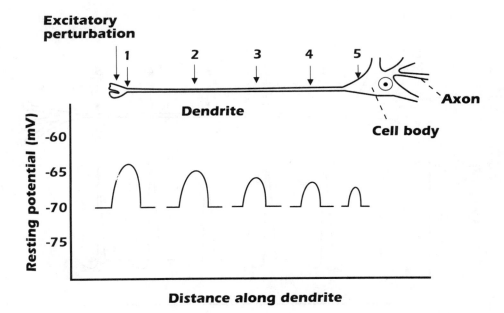

Figure 2–6. Graded potential following a perturbation showing how it decrements as it travels from the site of perturbation. Numbers 2 through 5 are sites of recording the decrementing graded potential.

potential. The action potential begins in the axon hillock or in the initial portion of the axon. There is a sudden opening of ion channels and a rapid flow of positive sodium ions into the cell. This initiates a wave of negativity that sweeps down the axon without decrementing all the way to the terminal boutons of the axon and its collaterals. This propagated wave of negativity is the action potential, also called the **nerve impulse** (Figure 2–7).

Because the nerve impulse maintains its full electrical charge the entire length of the axon, traveling from axon hillock to terminal bouton without decrement, it is called an **all-or-none phenomenon**. That is to say, at any given time along the axon, there is either an action potential or a resting potential; there is no in-between state.

D. Synaptic Transmission

When action potentials reach the terminal boutons, they activate the synaptic vesicles. The vesicles move to the

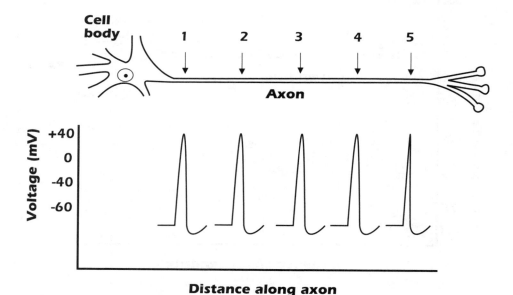

Figure 2–7. An action potential initiated at 1 does not decrement as it is propagated along the axon and recorded at sites 2, 3, 4, and 5. It is an all-or-none potential.

THE NEURONAL KISS

An easy way to visualize and remember the functions of a synapse is to think of it as a "neuronal kiss."

- It communicates information.
- It does not make a permanent commitment.
- It may be excitatory or inhibitory.

---

plasma membrane of the terminal bouton and release chemicals called **neurotransmitters** into the synaptic cleft.

There are many different neurotransmitters; each is found only in certain types of neurons, although a given type of neuron may have more than one neurotransmitter.

Neurotransmitters cause ion channels to open in the post-synaptic membrane of the next cell. Which ion channels are opened depends on which neurotransmitter is released. The ion channels in turn determine whether the next cell is excited (i.e., the resting potential is decreased) or inhibited (i.e., the resting potential is increased).

The next cell—that is, the cell on the other side of the synapse, which is affected by the neurotransmitter—may be a gland cell, a muscle cell, or another neuron. Excitation causes action: the gland cell secretes, the muscle cell contracts, the neuron sends action potentials along its axon— provided that the resting depolarization summates by (i.e., adds up to) about 15 mV at the axon hillock. Inhibition hyperpolarizes the cells so that they require greater excitatory stimulation for action.

Summary

At rest, all cells, including neurons, have a resting potential of about −70 mV. Perturbing the plasma membrane causes local (graded) potentials that decrement. Sufficient depolarization of a neuron initiates action potentials (nerve impulses), which are propagated the length of the axon without decrementing. At the terminal bouton, action potentials cause release of neurotransmitters into the synaptic cleft.

IV. SATELLITE CELLS

Although neurons are the principal cells of the nervous system and perform the information processing, the satellite cells, which facilitate the activity of the neurons, are actually more numerous. Satellite cells in the CNS are called **glial cells**; those in the PNS are called **Schwann cells**.

A. Oligodendroglia and Schwann Cells

Layers of the bilipid membranes of Schwann cells, and of a type of glial cells called **oligodendroglia**, wrap around axons and directly influence the propagation of nerve impulses; some axons have a single or very few layers, others have hundreds (Figure 2–8).

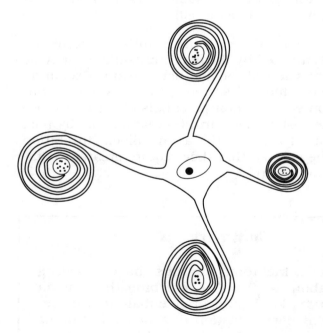

Figure 2–8. Schematic diagram of a Schwann cell (PNS) or oligodendrocyte (CNS) showing how extensions of its plasma membrane wrap around neuronal axons to form the myelin sheath.

1. Myelinated Axons

When more than one bilipid layer wraps around an axon, the layers form the axon's **myelin sheath**. The thicker an axon's myelin sheath, the more rapid the propagation of nerve impulses along it. Similarly, the larger the axon's diameter, the more rapid the propagation.

The myelin sheath extends all the way from the axon hillock to the telodendria or terminal boutons and is composed of extensions of the plasma membranes of many satellite cells, either Schwann cells (in the PNS) or oligodendroglia (in the CNS). The tiny space between one satellite cell and another is called a **node of Ranvier**. At these sites, where the axon is not covered by myelin, there are large concentrations of sodium channels in the axon's plasma membrane.

Action potentials are not propagated continuously along a myelinated axon; instead, they actually jump from the sodium channels at one node of Ranvier to those at the next. This is called **saltatorial** (jumping) **conduction** of the action potential. It is much more rapid than what occurs in unmyelinated axons.

2. Unmyelinated Axons

Unmyelinated axons are those wrapped with only a single layer of satellite cell membrane. They are always smaller than myelinated axons. Nerve impulses are propagated smoothly and continuously and, compared to myelinated axons, slowly along the axon's length.

B. Astrocytes

Astrocytes (star-shaped cells) are a second class of satellite cells (Figure 2–9). They are found only in the CNS; therefore, like oligodendroglia, they are glial cells. Unlike oligodendroglia, they do not produce myelin.

Astrocytes are scattered among neurons throughout the brain and spinal cord. They have many processes, which extend outward in a star-shaped pattern. They control the ionic environment of the extracellular fluid so that nerve

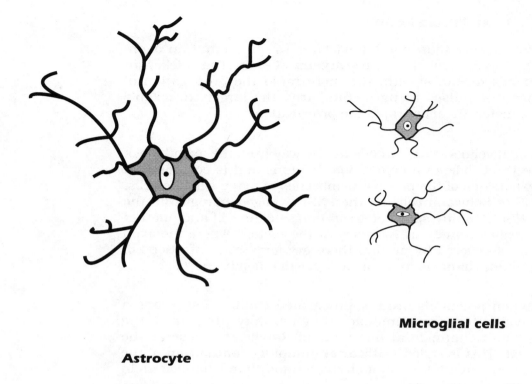

Microglial cells

Astrocyte

Figure 2–9. Diagrams of an astrocyte and two microglial cells.

cells can function optimally. Some processes contact blood capillaries and participate in controlling which chemicals pass between them and the extracellular space.

C. Microglia

Microglia form the final class of satellite cells; they are also found only in the CNS (Figure 2–9).

Microglia proliferate at the site of a brain or spinal cord injury in a process called **gliosis**. They form the equivalent of scar tissue and reduce damage to surrounding neurons. They are the only cells of the CNS that can reproduce themselves (divide) even when mature.

Microglia also function as the scavengers of the central nervous system, taking in and destroying worn-out or foreign materials.

Summary

The satellite cells of the PNS are Schwann cells; those of the CNS are glial cells, which are subdivided into oligodendroglia, astrocytes, and microglia. Satellite cells facilitate neurons. Schwann cells and oligodendroglia form the myelin sheaths of PNS and CNS neurons, respectively; myelin sheaths facilitate the propagation of action potentials. Astrocytes control the neuronal cells' environment; microglia assist in repair following brain damage.

V. DIVERSITY OF NEURONAL TYPES

Neurons are classified as **multipolar**, **bipolar**, or **unipolar**, depending on how many processes they have.

A. Multipolar Neurons

Multipolar neurons, the most numerous class, are highly diverse in both the length of their axons and the number, length, and branching patterns of their dendrites. Nevertheless, both functionally and structurally, all multipolar neurons belong to one of two types, and both types participate in circuits.

1. Projection Neurons: Golgi Type I

The first is the **Golgi type I**, or **projection neuron**. These are large neurons with long axons that, as the name indicates, project to distant portions of the nervous system (Figure 2–10). Some projection neurons have their cell bodies in the CNS and extend their axons into the PNS, where they innervate muscles or glands. Other projection neurons stay within the CNS and innervate (synapse with) other neurons.

2. Local Circuit Neurons: Golgi Type II

The second multipolar type is **the Golgi type II**, or **local circuit neuron**. These are usually small neurons in the CNS with short axons terminating on nearby neurons; they do not extend to distant parts of the nervous system or pass out to the peripheral nervous system. They integrate the functioning of neuronal groups in the CNS.

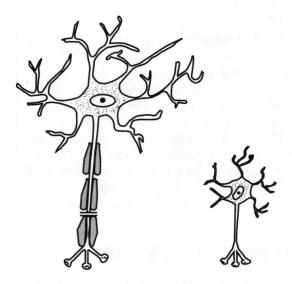

Projection neuron   **Local circuit neuron**

Figure 2–10. Diagrams of a projection neuron and a local circuit neuron. The gap in the myelinated axon of the projection neuron indicates the omission of a large length of the axon.

Note that neural information can sometimes be passed from one neuron to the next without nerve impulses.

Most local circuit neurons are unmyelinated. Some do not have action potentials, only graded potentials that cause release of neurotransmitters when they reach terminal boutons.

3. Circuits

Both projection and local circuit neurons are found in all three types of neural circuits:

- **motor circuits**, which control muscular activity or glandular secretions;
- **sensory circuits**, which receive and process information from sensory neurons in the periphery;
- **integrating circuits**, confined to the brain and spinal cord, which are neither primarily sensory nor primarily motor but concerned with synthesizing and refining neural information.

As a rule, the more complex the neuronal processing, the more local circuit neurons are present in such a circuit.

B. Bipolar Neurons

Some neurons are **bipolar** rather than multipolar. As the name implies, they have only two processes: one extends toward or into the periphery; the other extends toward or into the central nervous system. Both processes are usually unbranched (i.e., they have no collaterals).

Bipolar neurons are found in only four locations: in the retina of the eye, where they are one of several neuronal types; in the olfactory nerves; and in the auditory and vestibular portions of the vestibulocochlear nerve (cranial nerve VIII) (Figure 2–11).

Auditory and vestibular bipolar neurons are entirely myelinated—**peripheral process**, **central process**, and **cell body**. Their peripheral ends extend into the inner ear, where they synapse with sensory cells for hearing or vestibular function. Action potentials are propagated along their peripheral process, through the cell body, and then through the central process and into the brainstem to synapse on second order central auditory or vestibular neurons.

Note that both central and peripheral processes of auditory and vestibular bipolar neurons conduct and propagate nerve impulses and are called simply "processes." By contrast, in multipolar neurons, only axons propagate action potentials; their dendrites and cell bodies have only graded potentials.

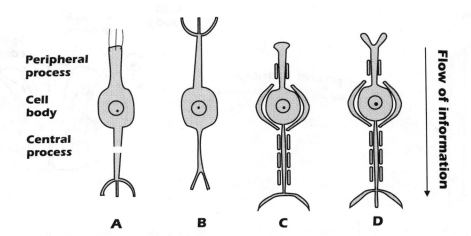

Figure 2–11. Schematic diagrams of bipolar neurons: **A**, a primary olfactory neuron; **B**, a bipolar retinal neuron; **C**, a primary auditory neuron; and **D**, a primary vestibular neuron.

C. Unipolar Neurons

There are also **unipolar neurons**. Their cell bodies lie in ganglia of the peripheral nervous system, just outside the central nervous system. They develop from bipolar neurons by fusing the portions of each process adjacent to the cell body, so that only one process leaves the cell body. A short distance from the cell body this single process divides into two processes: one goes out to peripheral portions of the body; the other goes centrally into the brain or spinal cord (Figure 2–12). Both the **peripheral process** and the **central process** may be myelinated or unmyelinated, and each can propagate nerve impulses. Because they develop from a bipolar predecessor, they are sometimes called **pseudo-unipolar**, meaning false unipolar neurons.

Because of this developmental similarity, unipolar neurons can be considered to be specialized bipolar neurons: both are primary sensory neurons.

Unipolar neurons carry sensory information from the periphery (e.g., from the skin) into the brain or spinal cord (Figure 2–12). They are called **primary sensory neurons** because they are the first neurons in a sensory pathway that eventually carries specific sensory information to areas of the cerebral hemisphere.

Excitation and inhibition occur at the tips of their peripheral processes, which have no satellite cells (Schwann cells) around them. If excitation causes sufficient depolarization there, action potentials will start where the Schwann cell covering begins. The action potentials are then propagated

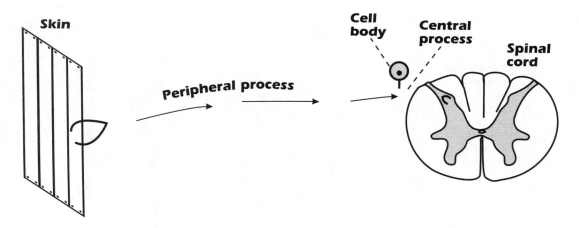

Figure 2–12. Diagram of a single unipolar neuron whose peripheral process extends to the skin. Its cell body is in a ganglion just outside the spinal cord and its central process extends into the spinal cord to synapse with neurons there.

in an all-or-none fashion along the peripheral processes to the central processes and along the central processes into the central nervous system. There, the central processes terminate; their terminal boutons synapse on groups of second order sensory neurons that analyze sensory information in the brain or spinal cord.

Note that, as in bipolar neurons, both the central and peripheral processes of unipolar neurons propagate action potentials. The central processes are structurally and functionally like axons of multipolar neurons because they also carry information away from the cell body; the peripheral processes propagate action potentials like axons, but carry information toward the cell body like dendrites.

Summary

Multipolar neurons can be subdivided into local circuit neurons (Golgi type II) and projection neurons (Golgi type I). These two types of neurons interact with each other during neuronal processing. Primary sensory neurons are either bipolar or unipolar. Both their peripheral and central processes propagate action potentials.

VI. NERVE-MUSCLE RELATIONSHIPS

While language is a function of the brain, speech is a motor activity that happens when the nervous system activates specific muscles. So we come now to a discussion of the general structure and function of **skeletal muscles** and the relationship of the nervous and muscular systems.

Note that all skeletal muscle contractions are motor activities.

A. Muscle and Muscle Cell Structure

There are three types of muscles: skeletal muscles (which move portions of the skeleton and are usually under voluntary control); **smooth muscles** (which cause smooth movements in intestines, blood vessels, etc., and are usually involuntary); and cardiac muscles (which pump blood from the heart). Like all organs, muscles are composed of cells.

Each type of muscle has its characteristic cells, but all are specialized to contract. We are concerned here with skeletal muscles, which are the only ones involved in speech.

1. Skeletal Muscles

Skeletal muscles are made up of large **skeletal muscle cells**, which attach to tendons, which in turn attach to bones or cartilages. Each skeletal muscle cell contains multiple nuclei and is packed with two types of contractile proteins, **actin** and **myosin**. These proteins are arranged parallel to one another so precisely that under the light microscope one can see stripes—the overlapping rows of myosin and actin molecules—at right angles to the long axis of the cells (Figure 2–13). This gives them the name **striated muscles**. When activated, the actin-myosin complex shortens, causing the cell to contract.

When a muscle contracts, its tone increases; when it relaxes, its tone decreases.

An individual muscle contains thousands of these large skeletal muscle cells, each of which is always in a state of either contraction or relaxation; there is no intermediate state between contracted and relaxed for individual cells. The degree of contraction for an entire muscle, called its **tone**, is determined by how many individual muscle cells are contracted and how many are relaxed at any given moment.

Under normal circumstances there is never a time when all the muscle cells of a given muscle are contracted. That situation is pathological, and is called **tetany**. Similarly, there is never a time when all the muscle cells of a muscle are relaxed. That happens only under deep anesthesia, when the muscle is said to be **flaccid**, or in a state of **flaccidity**.

2. Motor Units

Skeletal muscle cells are innervated by large multipolar neurons, called **alpha motor neurons.** Their somas lie in

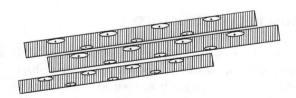

Figure 2–13. Three skeletal muscle cells, each with several nuclei and prominent striations caused by the orderly arrangement of actin and myosin molecules.

the brainstem or in the spinal cord; each axon extends out through peripheral cranial or spinal nerves and synapses on between 2 and 150 muscle cells (Figure 2–14).

A single alpha motor neuron and the muscle cells it innervates form a complex called a **motor unit**. "A motor unit of three" indicates an alpha motor neuron and the three muscle cells it innervates; "a motor unit of 120" indicates that this individual alpha motor neuron causes contractions in 120 muscle cells. The smaller the motor unit, the finer the control it exerts on the contraction of the muscle; the larger the motor unit, the grosser its control of a given muscle but the larger the increase in tone it produces. For example, the muscles that control your fingers have small motor units and fine dexterity. The large muscles that move your leg have large motor units and less precise control. Not surprisingly, the muscles that control your larynx, and thus much of your speech, have small motor units.

B. Proprioception

We are familiar with the fact that muscles *do* things. That is, they contract, or shorten, and cause parts of our body to move. In biological terms, these movements are **motor acts** controlled by alpha motor neurons.

Less familiar is the fact that muscles, tendons, and joints all contain small but important sense organs. Collectively

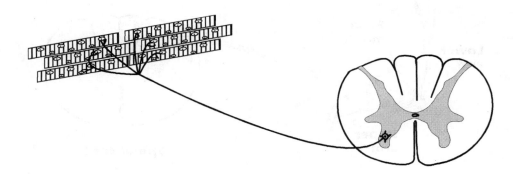

Figure 2–14. Diagram of a motor unit of 6. The single alpha motor neuron, whose cell body is in the spinal cord, extends its axon to the muscle and synapses with six skeletal muscle cells.

Much of the normal control of motor activity is determined by input from proprioceptors.

See the box on p. 54 for some fascinating details about muscle spindles.

called **proprioceptors**, their sensory nerves constantly send three kinds of information to the CNS: (1) the degree of stretch of each muscle; (2) the tension on each muscle; and (3) the position of each joint (Figure 2–15).

- The sense organs that respond to stretch are the **muscle spindles**. There are many tiny muscle spindles within each skeletal muscle. Stretching the muscle excites the muscle spindles; this initiates action potentials in their sensory nerves, which carry the information into the CNS.
- The sense organs that respond to tension are the **Golgi tendon organs**; they are found in all tendons—the fibrous connective tissue that attaches a muscle to a skeletal element (bone or cartilage). When a muscle contracts and increases its tone, or when it is pulled, the tension on the tendon is increased; this excites the Golgi tendon organs, whose sensory nerves send this information, via action potentials, to the CNS.
- The sense organs that respond to changes in the position of bones at a joint are called **joint receptors**. They are found in every moveable joint of the body (i.e., places where one bone or cartilage articulates with another in such a way that movement can occur). When the bones or cartilages of a joint move, the joint receptors respond to the change in pressure by initiating action potentials in their sensory nerves, which propagate the action potentials to the CNS.

Proprioception—the combined information from these three proprioceptor organs—keeps the CNS aware of all muscle

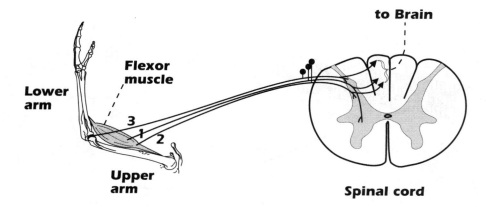

Figure 2–15. Three proprioceptive neurons sending information to the CNS: Neuron 1 from a muscle spindle; neuron 2 from a Golgi tendon organ; and neuron 3 from a joint receptor. All three project information to both the spinal cord for reflex activity and the brain.

activity and movement. In the CNS, this proprioceptive information is relayed both to alpha motor neurons and to higher nervous centers (e.g., the cerebellum and cerebrum), which then send their own action potentials to the alpha motor neurons. The final sum of excitation and inhibition on the alpha motor neurons determines the pattern of action potentials that are propagated along the axons of alpha motor neurons to the skeletal muscles.

Alpha motor neurons are also called **lower motor neurons**, in contrast to **upper motor neurons** whose cell bodies lie in the higher CNS centers and whose axons go to the lower motor neurons.

The axons of the lower motor neurons, or alpha motor neurons, form the *final common pathway*—so called because these axons carry action potentials to the skeletal muscles.

Summary

Skeletal muscles are composed of thousands of skeletal muscle cells. An alpha motor neuron and the skeletal muscle cells it innervates comprise a motor unit. Muscle tone is determined by the number of skeletal muscle cells contracted at a given moment. Muscles also have sense organs called proprioceptors; they are muscle spindles, Golgi tendon organs, and joint receptors. The information these proprioceptors send to the CNS helps in the control of all skeletal muscle activity.

VIII. WHAT HAS ALL THIS GOT TO DO WITH COMMUNICATION?

This brief tour through the cells of the nervous and skeletal muscle systems has given you an understanding of how they are built and how they function at a cellular level. This knowledge should enhance your appreciation of the systems most pertinent to communication scientists and clinicians. It is individual cells, working in concert with other cells, that produce the complex phenomena of hearing, speaking, using language, and maintaining balance and position.

MUSCLE SPINDLES

Within each skeletal muscle are several small sense organs called muscle spindles (Figure 2–16). They are often called **stretch receptors** because they detect any stretching of the muscle and send action potentials—via a unipolar neuron called an **annulospiral fiber** or **annulospiral neuron**)—to the CNS. The muscle spindles lie among the large skeletal muscle cells that are called **extrafusal muscle cells** (to distinguish them from the much smaller **intrafusal muscle cells**, which are found within each muscle spindle).

The muscle spindle's outer layer is fibrous connective tissue that connects the muscle spindle to the extrafusal muscle cells around it. Within this connective tissue covering are several small, specialized muscle cells called intrafusal muscle cells. Each intrafusal muscle cell attaches to the connective tissue capsule at each end. Intrafusal muscle cells are striated at each end but not striated in their central portion.

The terminal ends of peripheral fibers of large unipolar neurons, called annulospiral neurons, wrap around the nonstriated portion of the intrafusal muscle cells, synapsing with them. The cell body of the annulospiral neuron is located in a ganglion just outside the spinal cord or brainstem. Its central fiber enters the spinal cord or brainstem and forms an excitatory synapse with one or more alpha motor neurons. The axons of the alpha motor neurons leave the CNS and synapse with extrafusal muscle cells of the same muscle the muscle spindle is in.

Whenever a muscle is stretched, the muscle spindle's intrafusal muscle cells are also stretched, which causes them to excite the annulospiral neuron synapsing on them. This excitation is carried to the CNS via action potentials; thus the alpha motor neurons are excited to send action potentials to the extrafusal muscle cells, causing them to contract.

What results is a **stretch reflex**: when a muscle is stretched, lengthening it, the stretch reflex causes the muscle to contract just enough to bring it back to its original length. When a physician taps the tendon just under your knee cap and your leg slightly extends, he is testing your stretch reflex. Tapping the tendon stretches the tendon's muscle; the stretching excites the muscle spindles and causes action potentials in the annulospiral neurons; the action potentials excite alpha motor neurons, which causes the extrafusal muscle cells to contract.

Neurologists test a similar stretch reflex in the head—the **jaw jerk reflex**. Tapping the jaw stretches the muscles that close the jaw; the stretch reflex causes the jaw muscles to contact enough to bring the jaw back to position.

Interestingly, the CNS has motor neurons whose axons extend to, and synapse with, the striated portion of intrafusal muscle cells. These neurons are named **gamma motor neurons**. Their excitation is controlled by pathways originating in the brain. Excitation of the gamma motor neurons results in contractions of the intrafusal muscle cells. When contracted, the muscle cells shorten and thus increase the tension on the nonstriated portion of the intrafusal muscle cells. In this way the brain, via the gamma motor neurons, controls the sensitivity of the muscle spindles.

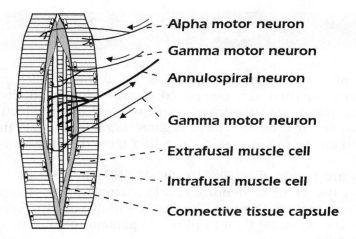

Alpha motor neuron
Gamma motor neuron
Annulospiral neuron
Gamma motor neuron
Extrafusal muscle cell
Intrafusal muscle cell
Connective tissue capsule

Figure 2–16. Diagram of a single muscle spindle between two extrafusal muscle cells. The stretch reflex involves the annulospiral neuron, carrying the stretch information from the muscle spindle to the CNS, and the alpha motor neuron, carrying the information to the extrafusal muscle cells and causing them to contract. The gamma motor neurons are controlled by the CNS and can cause the intrafusal muscle cells to contract, setting the sensitivity of the muscle spindle.

Understanding cell structure and function is thus a prerequisite to understanding both normal and abnormal communication systems. Throughout the remainder of this book you will be learning about the organization of the brain, about the structure and function of the vestibular and auditory systems, and about the speech and language systems.

CHAPTER 2 SUMMARY

All cells of the body are composed of small units called organelles which, in turn, are composed of four types of molecules: lipids, proteins, carbohydrates, and nucleic acids. Groups of cells form tissues; tissues form organs; organs form organ systems; and all the organ systems together form the organism.

Neurons are highly specialized cells. Multipolar neurons have a cell body, two or more dendrites, and a single axon. Axons end in swellings called terminal boutons which contain synaptic vesicles. The terminal bouton plus the plasma membrane of the adjacent cell is the synapse.

Nerve cells (like other cells) have an internal resting potential of about −70 mV. Perturbations of the plasma membrane cause local potentials (graded potentials) which may be excitatory (depolarization) or inhibitory (hyperpolarization). If the depolarization caused by local potentials summates to about −15 mV at the axon hillock, an action potential (nerve impulse) is initiated. The action potential is propagated along the axon without decrementing. At the terminal boutons, the action potentials cause release of neurotransmitters from the synaptic vesicles into the synaptic cleft. This in turn excites or inhibits the postsynaptic membrane, causing local potentials in the next cell.

Neurons are facilitated by satellite cells: Schwann cells in the PNS and glial cells in the CNS. Schwann cells (PNS) and oligodendroglia (CNS) form the myelin sheaths, which facilitate action potential propagation. Astrocytes control the extracellular environment of neurons and microglia help repair damage to the CNS.

Multipolar neurons may be either projection neurons (Golgi type I) or local circuit neurons (Golgi type II). Bipolar and unipolar neurons are both primary sensory neurons. They differ from multipolar neurons in that both their peripheral processes and central processes propagate action potentials.

Skeletal muscles are composed of huge numbers of skeletal muscle cells, each of which is capable of contraction. An alpha motor neuron and the skeletal muscle cells it innervates comprise a motor unit. Muscular activity is determined by the number of motor units active: the more motor units are active, the greater the muscle tone; conversely, the fewer are active, the less the muscle tone. Muscles contain three types of sense organs—muscle spindles, Golgi tendon organs, and joint receptors—which are collectively called proprioceptors. The input from these proprioceptors to the CNS is essential for both monitoring and controlling motor activity.

ADDITIONAL READING

Boyd, I. A., & Smith, R. S. (1994). The muscle spindle. In P. J. Dycke, P. K. Thomas, E. H. Lambert, & R. Bunge (Eds.), *Peripheral neuropathy* (Vol. 1, 2nd ed., pp. 171–202). Philadelphia: W. B. Saunders.

Burke, R. E. (1981). Motor units: Anatomy, physiology, and functional organization. In V. B. Brooks (Ed.), *Handbook of physiology. Section 1: The nervous system. Vol. II. Motor control* (Part 1, pp. 345–422). Bethesda, MD: American Physiological Society.

Jones, E. G. (Ed.). (1988). *Cell and tissue biology: A textbook of histology* (6th ed.) Baltimore, MD: Urban & Schwarzenberg.

Peters, A., Palay, S. L., & Webster, H. De F. (1991). *The fine structure of the nervous system: Neurons and their supporting cells* (3rd ed.) New York: Oxford University Press.

Schmidt, R. F. (1985). *Fundamentals of neurophysiology* (3rd rev. ed.). New York: Springer-Verlag.

STUDY GUIDE

Answer each question with a brief paragraph

1. What are proteins?
2. Describe the structure of the plasma membrane.
3. Describe the function of mitochondria.
4. What is the hierarchy from molecules to organisms?
5. How are nerve cells different from other cells of the body?
6. Describe the structure and function of synapses.
7. Compare and contrast local potentials and action potentials.
8. What are the functions of each type of satellite cell?
9. Compare and contrast bipolar neurons and unipolar neurons.
10. Describe a motor unit.
11. What is proprioception?
12. Describe a muscle spindle.

Odd One Out

In each of the following questions, choose the item that does not "fit" with the other three; briefly explain what the other three have in common that the odd one lacks. There may be more than one correct answer.

1. ____ ribosomes

   ____ carbohydrates

   ____ proteins

   ____ lipids

   WHY?

2. ___ collateral

   ___ telodendrion

   ___ dendrite

   ___ axon

   WHY?

3. ___ annulospiral neuron

   ___ unipolar neuron

   ___ bipolar neuron

   ___ multipolar neuron

   WHY?

4. ___ astrocytes

   ___ Schwann cells

   ___ oligodendroglia

   ___ microglia cells

   WHY?

5. ___ axon

   ___ dendrite

   ___ cell body

   ___ synapse

   WHY?

6. ___ Golgi tendon organ

   ___ skeletal muscle cell

   ___ muscle spindle

   ___ joint receptor

   WHY?

CHAPTER

3

GROSS ANATOMY AND BLOOD SUPPLY OF THE BRAIN

Learning neuroscience is not unlike learning a foreign language. First you must learn the vocabulary; then you can start using it.

The brain is an exceedingly complex organ whose surface abounds in irregular contours and structural landmarks. All have at least one name; some have more. Many names are of Latin or Greek derivation and are easier to remember if you know the root or English cognates; early anatomists liked to call them as they saw them, and some names are vivid in their imagery. Other names, alas, arise from placement, number, or the person who first described the structure (eponym).

The names must be learned before the significance of the structures can be discussed, so this chapter is heavy with terminology. Think of it as the gateway to more functional material to come.

As we embark on this lexicographer's adventure, keep in mind that, although the structures are separately named, they function not as separate entities but in concert. In fact, the separations between parts are often more arbitrary than functional.

In this chapter you will learn about:

- The membranes (meninges) covering the brain;
- The brain's four major divisions (brainstem, diencephalon, cerebellum, cerebrum);
- The surface anatomy and landmarks of each of these four parts;
- The blood vessels carrying blood to and from the brain.

I. MENINGES: THE BRAIN'S PROTECTION

Brain cells that are killed or injured cannot be replaced; lose a brain cell and it is gone for life. Because brain injury is permanent and brain tissue is delicate, protection of this organ is vital. The most obvious protector is the bony skull.

Less obvious but of great importance are three layers of membranes, called **meninges** (singular, meninx), and a layer of fluid, the **cerebrospinal fluid (CSF)**, which lies within them. (Meningitis is an inflammation of these membranes.) The outermost meninx, a tough, fibrous, leather-like membrane, is called the **dura mater** (Latin: tough mother). It adheres closely to the inner layer of the bones of the skull (Figure 3–1), except for two large extensions that

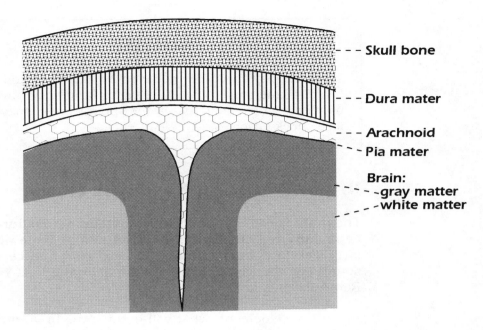

Figure 3–1. Relationship of the three meninges to the skull and brain. Note that the pia mater and part of the arachnoid extend into every groove of the brain but the dura mater does not.

penetrate crevices on the brain's surface: one of these extensions, the **falx cerebri**, extends down between the right and left cerebral hemispheres; the other, the **tentorium**, extends down between the cerebral hemispheres and the cerebellum. (More about these brain parts later.)

Adhering continuously to the inner surface of the dura mater, including the tentorium and falx cerebri, is the second of the three meninges, called the **arachnoid** (Latin: spider-like) layer. Web-like processes of the arachnoid extend toward the surface of the brain (Figure 3–1). Between these web-like processes is the **subarachnoid space**; it contains **cerebrospinal fluid (CSF)**, which acts like a shock-absorbing cushion.

The CSF not only acts as a shock absorber; it also provides a means of removing pathogens from the brain's environment.

The web-like extensions of the arachnoid are in contact with the third meninx, a thin, delicate layer called the **pia mater** (Latin: tender mother). The pia mater contains both large and small blood vessels and adheres tightly to the entire surface of the brain, following each groove and crevice.

Summary

The brain is physically protected by the skull and three layers of meninges: the dura mater, arachnoid, and pia mater. Cerebrospinal fluid in the subarachnoid space acts as a shock absorber.

II. MAJOR DIVISIONS OF THE BRAIN

The brain is composed of the **brainstem, cerebellum, diencephalon,** and **cerebrum**; the cerebrum is made up of two large **cerebral hemispheres**. (If cerebrum and cerebellum sound confusingly similar, see the following box, Hints for Remembering, for help.)

In early development, what will become the brain and spinal cord is a straight hollow tube filled with CSF. As development proceeds, the brain end of this neural tube grows faster than the spinal cord portion, making the brain much thicker than the spinal cord. This growth is greatest in the uppermost portion of the brain where the diencephalon and cerebrum form. In fact, the differential growth of these parts causes the straight neural tube to bend almost 90° at the junction of the brainstem and diencephalon. Because of this bending, or flexure, the major axis of the CNS, called the **neuraxis**, is in a horizontal plane in the diencephalon and cerebrum, and in a vertical plane in the rest of the CNS (Figure 3–2).

This makes some directional anatomical descriptions confusing. *Dorsal* is the direction away from the original straight neuraxis and toward the back of the developing embryo. After the flexure occurs, dorsal becomes superior to the neuraxis of cerebrum and diencephalon, but remains posterior to the neuraxis of spinal cord and brainstem. Similarly, *ventral* becomes inferior to the neuraxis of cerebrum and diencephalon, but remains anterior to the neuraxis of spinal cord and brainstem (Figure 3–2).

A. Brainstem

The brainstem is continuous with the spinal cord. Attached to its posterior surface is the cerebellum; attached to its rostral (superior) end is the diencephalon ("between brain").

HINTS FOR REMEMBERING

Cerebral or *cerebrum*, and *cerebellar* or *cerebellum* are frequently confused by students new to the terminology of neuroscience. The words have similar spellings and pronunciations. The structures each have hemispheres that give rise to large tracts, called peduncles, and are covered by an outer layer of gray matter, called cortex—either cerebellar or cerebral.

It may help to remember that a "cerebral person" is a "thinking person," and that the cerebrum is where thinking occurs.

Some etymology may also help:

Cerebrum is the Latin word for *brain*; *cerebellum* is the diminutive form, meaning *little brain*. Remember that cerebrum is the shorter word but by far the larger structure.

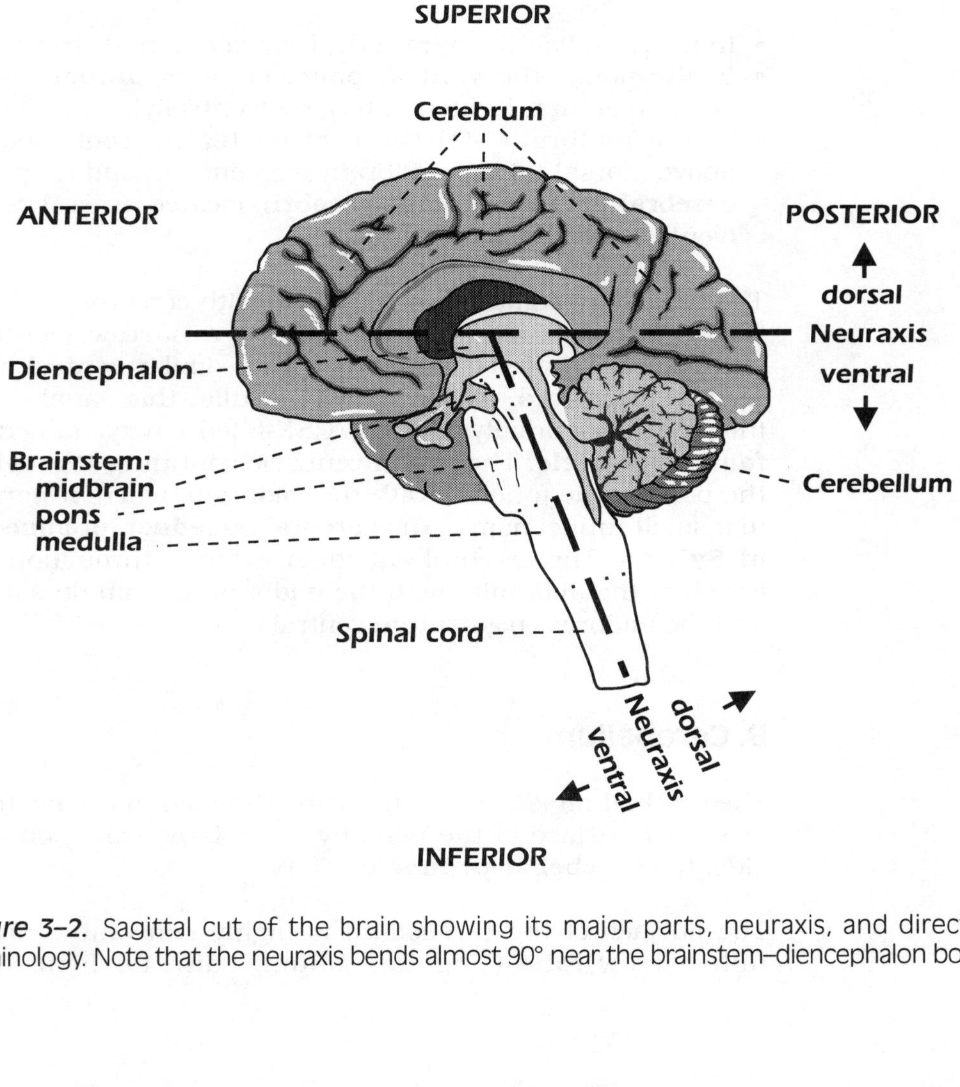

Figure 3–2. Sagittal cut of the brain showing its major parts, neuraxis, and directional terminology. Note that the neuraxis bends almost 90° near the brainstem–diencephalon border.

The brainstem is divided into three portions. The inferior portion, continuous with the spinal cord and, near their junction, indistinguishable from it, is the **medulla oblongata** (or **medulla**); the intermediate portion is the **pons**; the uppermost portion is the **midbrain**, which is continuous with the diencephalon.

The brainstem is also divided into **tegmental** and **nontegmental** portions (tegmentum is Latin for covering). The tegmentum, which forms its central core, is continuous throughout the brainstem: the tegmentum of the medulla is continuous superiorly with the tegmentum of the pons, which is continuous with the midbrain tegmentum (Figure 3–3).

The nontegmental portions of the brainstem are discontinuous, and are "tacked on," or appended to, the core's dorsal and ventral surfaces. They are (Figure 3–3):

- In the medulla—the **pyramids**, located anteriorly (ventrally).
- In the pons—the **ventral pons**, or **pons proper**, a very large structure, located anteriorly (ventrally).
- In the midbrain—(1) the **tectum** (Latin, roof), located above (dorsal to) the midbrain tegmentum; and (2) **paired cerebral peduncles (crus cerebri)**, located anterolaterally (ventrolaterally).

The brainstem contains cavities filled with cerebrospinal fluid (CSF). In the lower medulla there is a narrow, centrally located canal that is continuous with a similar **central canal** in the spinal cord. In the upper medulla, this canal dilates into a large, dorsally located, CSF-filled cavity named the **fourth ventricle**. The fourth ventricle continues throughout the pons to the junction with the midbrain, where it narrows to a small tunnel named the **cerebral aqueduct**, or **aqueduct of Sylvius**. The cerebral aqueduct extends throughout the length of the midbrain, with the midbrain tectum dorsal to it and the midbrain tegmentum ventral to it.

B. Cerebellum

The cerebellum is a large structure attached to the posterior or dorsal surface of the pons by three large tracts on each side, the **cerebellar peduncles**.

The surface of the cerebellum is highly convoluted due to tall, narrow **folia** (singular, folium; Latin for leaf). Each

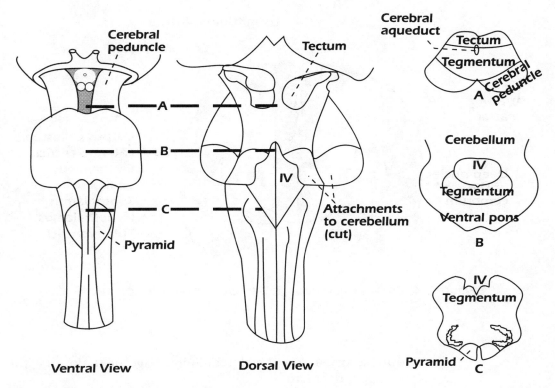

Figure 3–3. General features of brainstem organization. **A**, **B**, and **C** are cross-sections through the brainstem at levels indicated. IV = fourth ventricle.

folium is covered by three layers of gray matter that together are the **cerebellar cortex**. Central to the cortex there is a core of white matter that is continuous with the deep gray matter of the cerebellum.

C. Diencephalon

Rostral to the midbrain is the diencephalon, or "between brain"—so called because of its location between brainstem and cerebral hemispheres. It contains a tall, narrow, midline space filled with CSF—the **third ventricle**—which is continuous inferiorly with the cerebral aqueduct of the midbrain.

The diencephalon has four divisions (Figure 3–4):

- **thalamus**—the superior (dorsal) portion, largely obscured by cerebral hemispheres; the largest division;
- **hypothalamus**—the inferior (ventral) portion of the diencephalon; the second largest division;

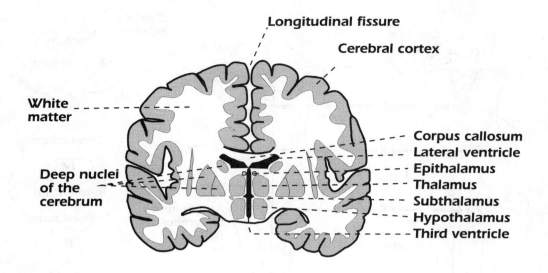

Figure 3–4. Cross-section through the cerebrum and diencephalon.

- **epithalamus**—on the dorsomedial edge of thalamus; the smallest division;
- **subthalamus**—between thalamus and hypothalamus, not reaching the surface; the second smallest division.

D. Cerebrum

During early development, the cerebral cortex is smooth. Because its surface grows faster than the skull, it must buckle in order to fit into its container, the braincase. This buckling forms the gyri and sulci.

The cerebrum is by far the largest part of the brain. It is comprised of two cerebral hemispheres. Although they develop as the rostral end of the neuraxis, they grow to such size that they come to lie not only rostral to the diencephalon but also dorsal, inferior, and lateral to it.

The surface of the cerebral hemispheres, like that of the cerebellum, is convoluted. It has **gyri** (singular, **gyrus**), which are broader than the folia of the cerebellum; between them are **sulci** (singular, **sulcus**), which are usually shallower than the grooves between cerebellar folia. A few sulci are so deep that they are called **fissures** instead of sulci. The **longitudinal fissure** is the deepest and longest; it lies between right and left cerebral hemispheres (Figure 3–4). The **transverse fissure**, almost as deep, separates the inferior surface of the cerebral hemispheres from the cerebellum.

Sheets of gray matter, the **cerebral cortex**, cover the surface of all the gyri and sulci of the cerebrum (Figure 3–4). Deep to the cerebral cortex lie broad sheets of white matter, and deep to these, large nuclei. The white matter is composed of large fiber tracts that connect the cerebral hemispheres with one another and the cerebral cortex with other parts of the CNS. The largest tract in the brain is the **corpus callosum**; it connects almost all parts of the cerebral cortex of one hemisphere to almost all parts of the cerebral cortex of the other hemisphere.

Each cerebral hemisphere also contains a large CSF-filled space, the **lateral ventricle**. Each lateral ventricle is connected with the midline third ventricle by a small opening called the **interventricular foramen** (Latin, hole; plural, foramina), or **foramen of Monro**.

E. Ventricular System

Thus the brain contains four ventricles. Starting rostrally, these are (Figure 3–5):

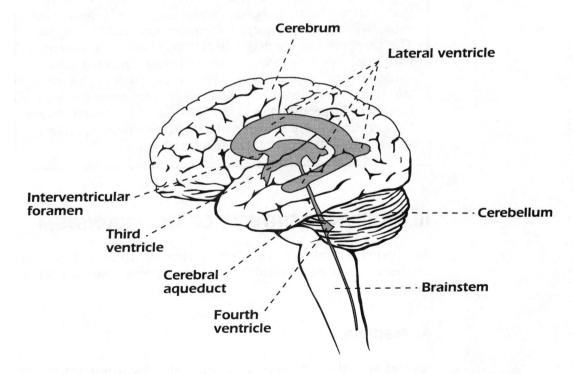

Figure 3–5. Lateral view of brain showing the ventricular system deep within.

- one **lateral ventricle** in each cerebral hemisphere;
- the **third ventricle** in the diencephalon; and
- the **fourth ventricle** in the pons and upper part of the medulla.

They are continuous with one another. The two lateral ventricles connect with the third ventricle by way of the foramina of Monro; the third connects with the fourth by way of the cerebral aqueduct (aqueduct of Sylvius) in the midbrain. The CSF in the ventricles is also continuous with that in the subarachnoid space through three openings in the roof of the fourth ventricle.

Summary

The brainstem (medulla, pons, and midbrain) is composed of a central core called the tegmentum plus nontegmental structures (pyramids, ventral pons, tectum, and cerebral peduncles). The cerebellum is attached to the posterior surface of the brainstem by cerebellar peduncles. The diencephalon has four parts: the thalamus, hypothalamus, epithalamus, and subthalamus. The cerebrum is divided into two cerebral hemispheres, which are composed of a convoluted cerebral cortex underlaid by white matter and large nuclei. The ventricular system, which is filled with cerebrospinal fluid, has four large divisions: the two lateral ventricles (in the cerebrum), the third ventricle (in the diencephalon), and the fourth ventricle (in the brainstem).

III. SURFACE ANATOMY OF THE BRAINSTEM

As described above, the brainstem is divided into the medulla (or medulla oblongata), the pons, and the midbrain.

A. Medulla

As the spinal cord passes through the **foramen magnum** (Latin: large hole) in the base of the skull, its name changes to the medulla of the brainstem. On the medulla's posterior surface are two large tracts, the **fasciculus gracilis** and **fasciculus cuneatus**, which are continuous with the same structures in the spinal cord (Figure 3–6). When these tracts reach the lower border of the fourth ventricle, their axonal endings synapse with large aggregates of neuronal cell bodies called, respectively, the **nucleus gracilis** and **nucleus cuneatus**. These nuclei are located in swellings—the **gracile tubercle** medially and the **cuneate tubercle** laterally—which mark the termination of the tracts. The inferior tip of the fourth ventricle, bordered by the gracile tubercle, is called the **obex**.

On the anterior (ventral) surface of the medulla, on each side of the midline, is a longitudinal swelling called the **pyramid**, which contains the **pyramidal tract**, or **corticospinal tract** (Figure 3–7). This tract is composed of axons passing from cell bodies in the cerebral cortex down to the spinal cord. The left and right pyramidal tracts cross each other in the lower part of the medulla; thus the output from the right side of the brain goes to the left side of the body and vice versa. The crossing point, called the **pyramidal decussation**, can be seen on the anterior surface of the medulla. Recall that the pyramids are the only nontegmental parts of the medulla.

"Pyramidal" is pronounced pi - rămd'l, not pi'- rămid'l

Just lateral and dorsal to the pyramid is a swelling called the **olive**, a prominent olive-shaped bulge caused by the underlying **inferior olivary nucleus**. In the groove between the olive and the pyramid are the rootlets of the XIIth cranial (**hypoglossal**) **nerve**. In the groove just above and lateral to the olive are rootlets of cranial nerves IX, X, and XI (**glossopharyngeal**, **vagus**, and **spinal accessory**) (Figure 3–7).

Three more cranial nerves attach to the brain at the rostral-most portion of the medulla where it abuts the pons. The rootlets of the VIth cranial nerve (**abducens**) are attached just lateral to the pyramid where it emerges from the pons. Cranial nerves VII and VIII (**facial** and **vestibulocochlear**) are attached more laterally, in an area called the **cerebellopontine angle**, where the pons, medulla, and cerebellum come together. Where the VIIIth nerve attaches to the brainstem there is a small mass of gray matter, the **dorsal cochlear nucleus**, which causes a surface swelling called the **acoustic tubercle** (Figure 3–6).

It is here at the cerebellopontine angle that acoustic neuromas sometimes form on the VIIIth nerve.

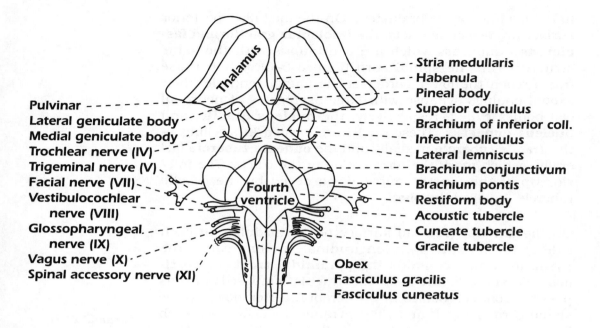

Figure 3–6. Dorsal view of brainstem and diencephalon after removal of cerebrum and cerebellum.

B. Pons

The anterior surface of the pons proper is a large bulging mass of white matter that is composed of myelinated axons leaving the pons proper. These axons form the **middle cerebellar peduncle**, or **brachium pontis** (Latin, arm of the pons), and enter the cerebellum (Figure 3–7). They carry information to the cerebellum.

There are two other cerebellar peduncles; they carry information both to and from the cerebellum. The lowermost is the **inferior cerebellar peduncle**, or **restiform body**. The uppermost is the **superior cerebellar peduncle**, or **brachium conjunctivum**.

When the cerebellum has been dissected from the brainstem, one can see the cut surfaces of these three peduncles (Figure 3–6). They border each side of the floor of the fourth ventricle, which forms the posterior surface of the pons.

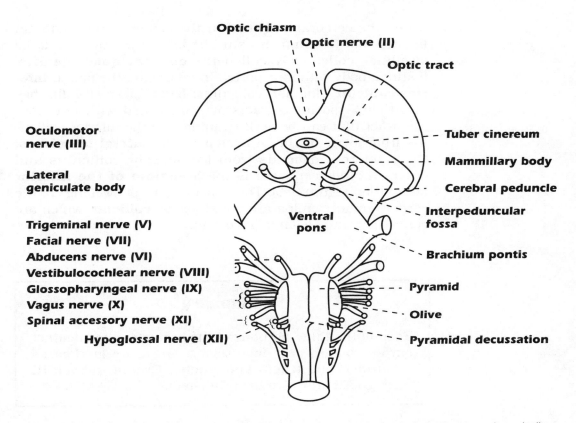

Figure 3–7. Ventral view of brainstem and diencephalon after removal of cerebrum and cerebellum.

Two cranial nerves attach to the pons. Cranial nerve V (**trigemina**l) attaches to the ventrolateral surface of the pons proper (Figures 3–6 and 3–7); cranial nerve IV (**trochlear**) attaches to the dorsal (posterior) surface at the midbrain-pons junction (Figure 3–6).

C. Midbrain

In the midbrain there are cerebral (rather than cerebellar) peduncles, sometimes called the crus cerebri (Latin: leg of the cerebrum). They are large swellings on either side of the anterior lateral aspect of the midbrain. Between them is a deep depression, the **interpeduncular fossa** (*inter*, between; *fossa*, depression). Cranial nerve III (**oculomotor**) emerges from the interpeduncular fossa (Figure 3–7).

Above the cerebral aqueduct in the center of the midbrain lies its roof (tectum). Its surface is marked by four large swellings collectively called the **corpora quadrigemina** (Latin: a body with four parts). Inferiorly are the paired **inferior colliculi** (singular, colliculus; Latin for small hill); they and their associated tracts are concerned with audition. The tract that can be seen running into the inferior colliculus from lower in the brainstem is the **lateral lemniscus**; the tract that ascends from the inferior colliculus and enters the diencephalon is the **brachium of the inferior colliculus** (Figure 3–6). The superior pair of swellings of the corpora quadrigemina are the **superior colliculi**, which are concerned with vision (Figure 3–6).

Summary

Each of the three portions of the brainstem has distinct surface bulges and depressions which are landmarks for underlying tracts and nuclei. Cranial nerves III through XII attach to the brainstem.

IV. SURFACE ANATOMY OF THE DIENCEPHALON

This partial crossing of fibers, which feeds information from the right and the left eyes to the same part of the brain, is the anatomical basis for stereoscopic vision.

A portion of the hypothalamus forms the inferior surface of the diencephalon. Anteriorly are the right and left **optic nerves** (cranial nerve II); the **optic chiasm**; and, extending dorsolaterally, the **optic tracts** (Figure 3–7). About half of the optic nerve fibers enter the optic tract of the same side; the other half cross the midline in the optic chiasm and enter the optic tract on the opposite side.

Just behind the optic chiasm is a swelling called the **tuber cinereum**, to which is attached the **pituitary gland**. Behind the tuber cinereum are two small swellings, one on either side of the midline, called the **mammillary bodies** (Figure 3–7).

A sagittal section of the diencephalon passes through the center of the third ventricle (see Figure 3–10 in section VI) and reveals its continuity with the other ventricles: the lateral ventricles anteriorly (via the foramina of Monro); and the cerebral aqueduct of the midbrain posteriorly.

In the lateral aspect of the third ventricle there is a shallow groove called the **hypothalamic sulcus**. Ventral to that sulcus, the third ventricle lines the hypothalamus; dorsal to it, the third ventricle lines the thalamus. Frequently, however, a portion of the thalamus grows across the third ventricle, making the right and left halves of the thalamus continuous. This continuity, when it occurs, is called the **massa intermedia** or **interthalamic adhesion**.

The thalamus is the largest structure of the diencephalon. It extends posteriorly and partially overlies the midbrain tectum with a portion called the **pulvinar**. Two thalamic swellings bulge out inferior to the pulvinar. The medial swelling is the **medial geniculate body**, at the end of the brachium of the inferior colliculus (Figure 3–6). Lateral to it is the **lateral geniculate body**, at the end of the optic tract (Figure 3–7).

The epithalamus is a narrow structure that lies along the dorsomedial border of the thalamus at the dorsal edge of the third ventricle. It is made up of a tract, the **stria medullaris**, which goes posteriorly to a nucleus, the **habenula**. Short tracts go from the habenula to a midline structure, the **pineal body**. These structures—stria medullaris, habenula, and pineal body—comprise the entire epithalamus (Figure 3–7).

So parts of three of the four portions of the diencephalon can be seen from the surface: the hypothalamus, the thalamus, and the epithalamus. The subthalamus is not a surface structure.

Recall that a sagittal section passes through the midline, dividing a structure into equal right and left halves.

Summary

Only small parts of the diencephalon form surface structures. However, these bulges and depressions are distinct landmarks for underlying structures. Cranial nerve II (optic nerve) attaches to the diencephalon.

EPITHALAMUS: SEAT OF THE SOUL?

We'll not be discussing the epithalamus in the remainder of this text, because, to the best of our knowledge, it has nothing to do with speech, language, balance, or hearing. In fact, we know embarrassingly little about its functioning, particularly in humans. In some amphibians and reptiles it forms a "third eye:" a light-sensitive, midline organ. In the same animals—chameleons, for instance—it controls color changes in the skin.

The pineal body, a midline structure in the brain, has fascinated both scientists and philosophers for centuries. In the 17th century, the scientist-philosopher René Descartes, a mechanist, suggested, perhaps facetiously, that the pineal is the seat of the soul: in its midline position, it could sway to the right, and then to the left, sending its "vital ethers of the soul" first to one hemisphere and then to the other. From the cerebral hemispheres, nerve fibers could carry the vital ethers throughout the body.

In the centuries since Descartes, we still have not found a satisfactory explanation of the function(s) of the pineal.

V. SURFACE ANATOMY OF THE CEREBELLUM

The surface of the cerebellum is characterized by many tall, narrow **folia** composed of white matter overlaid by gray matter. A sagittal cut through the cerebellum shows the depth of the sulci between the folia and the white matter that underlies the cortex at the core of each folium (Figure 3–8). In such a view, the white matter forms a distinctive, finely branching pattern. It is sometimes called the **arbor vitae** ("tree of life"—also the name of a group of cedar trees with complex branching leaves).

The cerebellum can be divided into three lobes: a relatively small **anterior lobe**, a large **posterior lobe**, and a very small inferior **flocculonodular lobe** (Figure 3–8B). Alternatively, the cerebellum can be divided into a midline portion called the **vermis** and two large, lateral swellings off the vermis called the **cerebellar hemispheres** (Figure 3–8A).

Deep within the white matter of the cerebellum are four large nuclei, the **deep nuclei of the cerebellum**. The axons

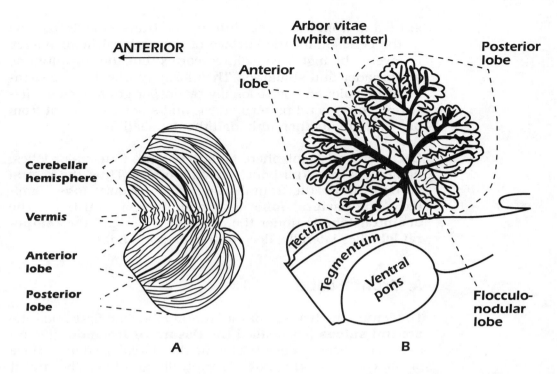

Figure 3–8. **A**. Superior view of cerebellum. **B**. Sagittal section through cerebellum.

of these nuclei carry information from the cerebellum to the brainstem via the restiform body and the brachium conjunctivum—two of the three (on each side) cerebellar peduncles.

Summary

The cerebellum can be divided into an anterior lobe, posterior lobe, and flocculonodular lobe. Alternatively, it can be divided into a midline vermis and the lateral cerebellar hemispheres.

VI. SURFACE ANATOMY OF THE CEREBRUM

The cerebrum is made up of the two cerebral hemispheres. They are separated from one another by the longitudinal fissure, and from the cerebellum by the transverse fissure. As in the cerebellum, the surface of the cerebral hemispheres is covered by highly convoluted cortex; but the convolutions are broader and shallower. They form gyri, which are separated by sulci and occasionally by deeper grooves called fissures. The general pattern of gyri and sulci is constant from one brain to another, although the details differ.

Each cerebral hemisphere is divisible into four major lobes, named for the skull bones they lie under. Thus the rostral portion, under the frontal bone, is the **frontal lobe**. Similarly, the **parietal lobe** lies under the parietal bone; the **occipital lobe** is under the occipital bone; and the **temporal lobe** lies laterally, deep to the temporal bone.

A. Frontal Lobe

To identify the borders of the frontal lobe, one first finds the **central sulcus** (also called the **fissure of Rolando**) (Figure 3–9). This deep groove begins at the dorsal medial surface of the cerebrum and extends ventrally and laterally until it ends at the even deeper **lateral sulcus** (also called the **lateral fissure** or **Sylvian fissure**). All of the cerebrum that lies anterior to the central sulcus and above the lateral sulcus makes up the frontal lobe (Figure 3–9).

The large gyrus just in front of the central sulcus is called the **precentral gyrus**. It contains the **primary motor cortex**, which also extends onto the medial surface of the hemisphere where it is called the anterior part of the **paracentral lobule** (Figure 3–10).

Although described solely by their anatomy, these areas are also important for their distinct functional identities.

Although the cerebral cortex is always composed of several (usually six) layers of neurons, microscopic examination shows that, from one area of the brain to another, these layers differ in thickness and in the proportions of neuronal types they contain. These differences were first described in detail in the human brain in 1909 by **Korbinian Brodmann**. He assigned a number to each distinct part of the cerebral cortex he identified, and some of those designations are still important for speech, hearing, and language professionals to know. In the frontal lobe:

- The **primary motor cortex**, including the precentral gyrus and the anterior part of the paracentral lobule, is **Brodmann's area 4**.

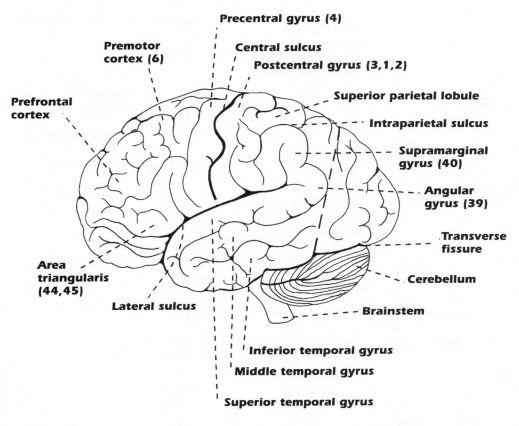

Figure 3–9. Lateral view of brain showing cerebral landmarks. The dashed line from the top of the parieto-occipital sulcus to the preoccipital notch shows the boundary between parietal and occipital lobes (upper part) and between the temporal and occipital lobes (lower part).

- Just in front of the precentral gyrus, in the dorsolateral portion of the frontal lobe and not extending to the lateral fissure, is the **premotor cortex, Brodmann's area 6**.
- Inferiorly, near the edge of the frontal lobe at the lateral fissure, is an area called the **area triangularis, Brodmann's areas 44 and 45** (Figure 3–9). On one side only (usually the left), this area controls expressive speech and is called **Broca's area**, in honor of **Paul Broca** who first determined its functional significance.
- The portion of the frontal lobe in front of the area triangularis and the premotor cortex (which contains several of Brodmann's areas) is called the **prefrontal cortex** (Figure 3–9).

On the inferior surface of the frontal lobe is a distinct tract, the **olfactory tract**; at its rostral end is a swelling of gray matter, the **olfactory bulb** (Figure 3–11). The **olfactory nerve**

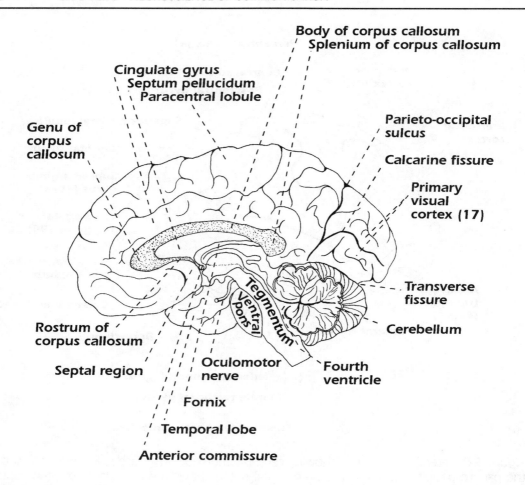

Figure 3–10. Sagittal view of brain showing cerebral landmarks. The corpus callosum's cut edge is stippled.

(cranial nerve I) enters directly into the olfactory bulb. These structures carry and process olfactory (smell) information.

B. Parietal Lobe

Immediately behind the frontal lobe is the parietal lobe. On the medial surface of the brain it is easy to identify the posterior boundary of the parietal lobe, which separates it from the occipital lobe. It is a deep sulcus named the **parieto-occipital sulcus** (Figure 3–10). No such division is seen on the lateral surface, where you must use your imagination to determine the border between the parietal and occipital lobes. Imagine a line from the top of the parieto-occipital sulcus down to a small notch, the **preoccipital notch**, on

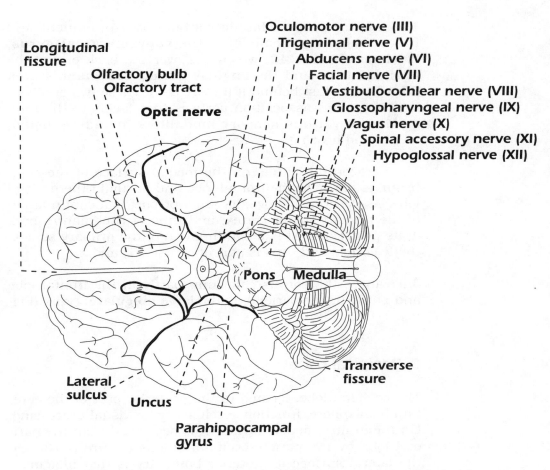

Figure 3–11. Inferior view of brain showing cerebral landmarks and cranial nerves.

the inferior surface of the hemisphere. This imaginary line separates the parietal and occipital lobes dorsally, and the occipital and temporal lobes ventrally (Figure 3–9).

A large gyrus borders the central sulcus in the parietal lobe. It is called the **postcentral gyrus**, and it is the **primary somesthetic cortex** (Figure 3–9). Somesthetic means sensory for proprioception, touch, pressure, temperature, and pain. This postcentral gyrus comprises **Brodmann's areas 3, 1, and 2**—always named in that order for historical reasons.

The remainder of the parietal lobe is divided by a sulcus, frequently incomplete, which is posterior to the postcentral gyrus and is called the **intraparietal sulcus**. Above this sulcus lies the **superior parietal lobule**; below it, the **inferior parietal lobule** (Figure 3–9).

The inferior parietal lobule contains two prominent and functionally significant gyri: the **supramarginal gyrus**, **Brodmann's area 40**, which lies over the back end of the lateral sulcus; and the **angular gyrus, Brodmann's area 39**, which is just behind it (Figure 3–9). These two gyri contain important association cortices that facilitate the integration of various sensory modalities including vision, touch, and hearing.

The paracentral lobule, on the medial surface of the cerebrum, is partly in the frontal lobe and partly in the parietal lobe. As described above, its anterior part is a continuation of the primary motor cortex, and thus of Brodmann's area 4; its posterior part is a continuation of the primary somesthetic cortex, and thus is part of areas 3, 1, and 2.

Just above the corpus callosum, partly in the frontal lobe and partly in the parietal, is the large **cingulate gyrus** (Figure 3–10).

C. Occipital Lobe

The occipital lobe, located in the posterior part of the cerebral hemisphere, functions exclusively for visual processing. On the brain's medial surface it is separated from the parietal lobe by the parieto-occipital sulcus (Figure 3–10). On the lateral surface its anterior boundary is that imaginary line from the top of the parieto-occipital sulcus to the preoccipital notch (Figure 3–9). The prominent sulcus on the medial surface of the occipital lobe is the **calcarine fissure**. The gyri just above and just below the calcarine fissure together form the **primary visual cortex, Brodmann's area 17** (Figure 3–10). The remainder of the occipital lobe (both medially and laterally) is made up of **association visual cortices, Brodmann's areas 18 and 19**.

D. Temporal Lobe

The temporal lobe contains the cerebral cortex that is below the lateral sulcus and in front of that imaginary line between the parieto-occipital sulcus and the preoccipital notch. On the lateral surface, the temporal lobe consists of three long gyri: the **superior temporal gyrus**, the **middle temporal gyrus**, and the inferior **temporal gyrus** (Figure

3–9). The posterior two-thirds of the superior temporal gyrus on one side (usually the left) is the receptive speech association cortex, which functions to decode speech. It is **Wernicke's area**, named for **Carl Wernicke**, who first described its functional characteristics. On both right and left sides, this portion of the superior temporal gyrus is also part of **Brodmann's area 22** which, as we will discuss, extends onto the superior surface of the temporal lobe.

There is also an extensive cortex that can be seen only by spreading open the lateral fissure and looking down at the superior surface of the temporal lobe. There one sees one, two, or three prominent gyri; they are the **transverse gyri of Heschl** and the number varies from brain to brain and from side to side (Figure 3–12). This is the location of the **primary auditory cortex**, **Brodmann's areas 41 and 42**, which will be described in greater detail in Chapter 8.

The number of transverse gyri of Heschl has no known functional correlate.

Just behind the transverse gyri of Heschl there is a relatively flat area of the superior surface of the temporal lobe. This is the **planum temporale**—a continuation of area 22 on both sides and of Wernicke's area on (usually) the left side (Figure 3–12).

On the inferior surface of the temporal lobe, medial to the inferior temporal gyrus, is the large **parahippocampal gyrus**. Posteriorly it is continuous with the cingulate gyrus. Its most medial aspect, where it juts out toward the hypothalamus, is the **uncus** (Figure 3–11).

E. Insula

Insula is Latin for island and neuroanatomic for an isolated group of gyri, separate from the frontal, parietal, occipital, and temporal lobes. The insula (the collective term for the group) is located by spreading open the edges of the lateral sulcus and looking past the transverse gyri of Heschl and the planum temporale of the temporal lobe (Figure 3–12).

The insular cortex does not belong to any of the four major lobes of the cerebrum.

F. Sagittal Surface of the Cerebrum

A sagittal cut through the brain severs the corpus callosum (and all other crossing structures) at the midline and exposes the full extent of this massive tract that connects right and left cerebral cortices (Figure 3–10). The corpus

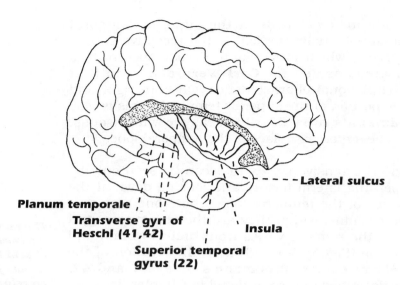

Planum temporale

Transverse gyri of
Heschl (41,42)

Superior temporal
gyrus (22)

Lateral sulcus

Insula

Figure 3–12. Lateral view of cerebrum with the portion of the frontal and parietal lobes above the lateral sulcus cut off. This cut allows a view of the insula and superior surface of the temporal lobe with the transverse gyri of Heschl and the planum temporale.

callosum (Latin: hard body) is thickest in its posterior part, which is called its **splenium** (Greek, bandage). Just in front of the splenium, where it narrows, is the **body of the corpus callosum**. Most anteriorly, the corpus callosum makes a 180° bend inferiorly; the bend is called the **genu of the corpus callosum** (Latin, knee, as in genuflect). The corpus callosum then extends posteriorly for a short distance, paralleling its body; this portion is called the **rostrum of the corpus callosum** (Latin, beak). The cerebral cortex that lies just below the rostrum of the corpus callosum is called the **septal region** (Figure 3–10).

A large fiber tract is seen arcing under the body of the corpus callosum toward the foramen of Monro; it is the **fornix**. A thin membrane runs between the fornix and the corpus callosum and forms part of the medial wall of the lateral ventricle; it is the **septum pellucidum** (Figure 3–10).

Where the fornix passes the foramen of Monro there is a small, transversely oriented tract called the **anterior commissure**. It connects the anterior-most parts of the right and left temporal cortices (Figure 3–10).

Summary

Each cerebral hemisphere has four major lobes (frontal, parietal, occipital, and temporal). Their surfaces are composed of cerebral cortices with gyri (convolutions) and sulci (grooves). The cerebral cortex is divided into many areas by both structural and functional criteria. Many of these areas are classified by a numbering system based on descriptions made by Brodmann in the early 20th century. Cranial nerve I (the olfactory nerve) attaches to the cerebrum.

VII. BLOOD SUPPLY

The brain requires a constant blood supply. Neurons have high metabolic rates and do not store energy reserves in the form of glycogen. The blood system brings carbohydrates (sugars) and the oxygen required to release the energy they carry. If the blood supply is interrupted, nerve cells do not receive these needed nutrients. They then die and are not replaced. It is important to understand the pattern of the brain's normal blood supply in order to interpret the results of, and possible therapies for, vascular accidents.

A blockage of a brain blood vessel, or bleeding from one, is called a cerebrovascular accident (CVA) or—more commonly—a stroke.

The brain receives blood through two arterial systems:

- The paired **vertebral arteries** travel up the neck, protected by the cervical vertebrae, and enter the cranial cavity at the foramen magnum.
- The paired **common carotid arteries** pass up through the neck and give off bilateral **internal carotid arteries**. The internal carotids enter the cranial cavity at the level of the hypothalamus. They are larger and carry more blood than the vertebral arteries.

A. Vertebral Arteries: Distribution and Branching

After they pass through the foramen magnum, the two vertebral arteries lie on the anterior (ventral) surface of the medulla (Figure 3-13). Each gives off a large branch, the **posterior inferior cerebellar artery**, which brings blood to part of the medulla and to the posterior inferior portion of the cerebellum. The two vertebral arteries then join, forming the midline **basilar artery** (Figure 3–13).

The basilar artery gives off two pairs of large branches: the **anterior inferior cerebellar arteries** and the **superior cerebellar arteries**.

The anterior inferior cerebellar arteries supply parts of the medulla and pons and the anterior inferior portion of the cerebellum (Figure 3–13). The **labyrinthine artery**, which may be a branch of the basilar artery or, frequently, a branch of the anterior inferior cerebellar artery, carries blood to both the cochlear and vestibular portions of the inner ear.

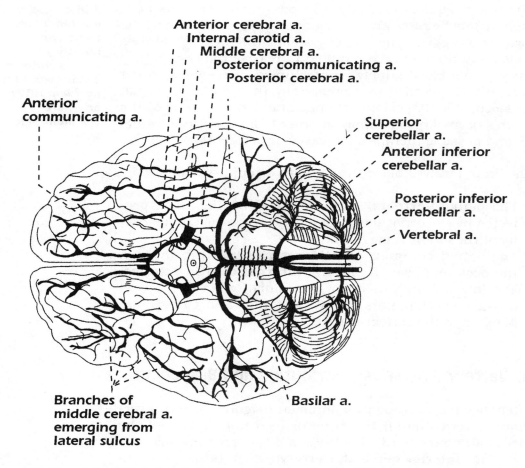

Figure 3–13. Inferior view of brain showing its arterial supply. a. = artery.

The superior cerebellar arteries supply the entire superior surface of the cerebellum.

Both the vertebral and basilar arteries also give off small arteries that go to immediately adjacent portions of the medulla and pons.

The basilar artery terminates at the upper level of the pons, where it bifurcates into two **posterior cerebral arteries**; these arteries carry blood up to the posterior portions of the cerebral hemispheres, primarily the occipital lobes (Figure 3–13).

B. Internal Carotid Arteries: Distribution and Branching

As the internal carotid arteries enter the cranial cavity, each gives off a small **posterior communicating artery,** which passes posteriorly and joins the posterior cerebral artery (Figure 3–13). The internal carotids also give off small **ophthalmic arteries**, which follow the optic nerves to the retina of the eye.

The largest portion of each internal carotid artery continues into the lateral sulcus as the **middle cerebral artery** (Figure 3–13). Just before entering the lateral sulcus, each middle cerebral artery gives off a slightly smaller branch, the **anterior cerebral artery** (Figure 3–13).

1. Middle Cerebral Artery

As each middle cerebral artery courses in the lateral sulcus it gives off many branches. Some go to large areas of the lateral surface of the cerebral hemisphere, including the lateral surfaces of the frontal, parietal, and temporal lobes (Figure 3–14). Others go into the deep substance of the cerebral hemispheres and diencephalon.

2. Anterior Cerebral Artery

The anterior cerebral arteries course along the medial surface of the cerebral hemisphere, going anterior to, and then superior to, the corpus callosum. Their branches go to the medial surfaces of the frontal and parietal lobes (Figure

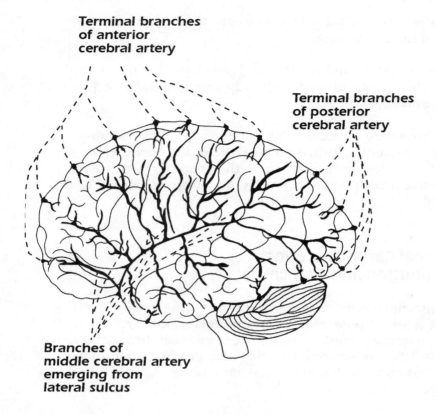

**Terminal branches
of anterior
cerebral artery**

**Terminal branches
of posterior
cerebral artery**

**Branches of
middle cerebral artery
emerging from
lateral sulcus**

Figure 3–14. Lateral view of the brain showing multiple branches of the middle cerebral artery emerging from the lateral sulcus and supplying most of the lateral surface of the cerebrum. Only distal ends of the anterior and posterior cerebral arteries reach the peripheral lateral surfaces of the cerebrum.

3–15). Before reaching the medial surface of the hemisphere, the two anterior cerebral arteries are interconnected by a small **anterior communicating artery**, which runs from one anterior cerebral artery to the other (Figure 3–13).

C. Arterial Circle of Willis

Details of the circle of Willis vary greatly from one brain to another.

On the brain's inferior surface, between the anterior region of the hypothalamus and the rostral edge of the pons, one can discern a roughly circular arrangement of interconnected arteries. It is called the **circle of Willis**, named for Thomas Willis, a seventeenth century anatomist and physician (Figure 3–13). Starting at the back of the circle, its components are:

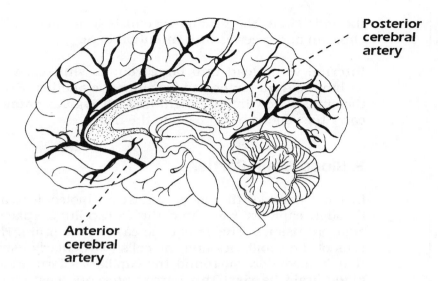

Figure 3–15. Medial view of brain showing distribution of the anterior and posterior cerebral arteries to the medial cerebrum. Note that branches of these arteries extend over the midline to the lateral surface of the cerebrum.

- the posterior cerebral arteries, as they form from the midline basilar artery;
- the posterior communicating arteries;
- the internal carotid arteries;
- the anterior cerebral artery, which comes off the middle cerebral artery as it forms from the internal carotid;
- the anterior communicating artery, which connects the two anterior cerebral arteries.

Thus the circle of Willis joins the arterial supply of the brain's two arterial systems—the vertebral and the internal carotids. Such connections between blood vessels, particularly between arteries, are called **anastomoses**. An anastomosis is a functional adaptation that provides an alternate vascular route to vital organs in case an artery is blocked. Blood can flow in either direction in these anastomoses, depending on where the blood pressure is greater.

D. Venous Drainage of the Brain

Fewer vascular accidents occur in the brain's venous system than in its arterial system, primarily because blood pressure is much lower in veins. Therefore, while vital to the individual, the venous system is less important to the clinician and receives little attention here.

Internal veins lead into large venous sinuses, which lie within the dura mater and flow into one another. Eventually the sinuses flow into the right and left **jugular veins**, which carry the venous blood back to the heart.

E. Blood-Brain Barrier

In most parts of the body, almost all molecules can pass through capillary walls into the extracellular space of the adjacent tissues. This is not the case in the brain. Here the cells of the capillaries and the cells (particularly astrocytes) that immediately surround the capillaries form a selective **blood-brain barrier**. This barrier prevents most pathogens, including most bacteria and viruses, from leaving the bloodstream and entering the brain. It also limits or eliminates the effects of many drugs on the brain. A notable exception, of course, are hallucinogenic drugs.

F. Cerebrospinal Fluid (CSF)

This includes the subarachnoid space along the spinal cord. A "lumbar tap" is a procedure that samples CSF from the lower spinal cord region so that its content can be analyzed.

Cerebrospinal fluid (CSF) is a clear, watery fluid containing almost no cells. It fills the subarachnoid space and bathes the entire central nervous system, and is found throughout its ventricles and other cavities (Figure 3–5).

CSF, a filtrate of blood, is formed by complex capillary networks lying within each of the four ventricles. The process, which is constantly ongoing, allows the clear plasma of the blood to pass through the capillary walls and holds back the blood cells and larger molecules.

Among other functions, CSF cleanses the central nervous system. It flows slowly but constantly through the ventricular system, exiting into the subarachnoid space through small apertures in the roof of the fourth ventricle. It is ultimately resorbed into the blood through specializations in the walls of the venous sinuses within the dura mater.

The system works well unless there is a blockage at a narrow spot—for instance, at the foramen of Monro, the cerebral aqueduct, or the apertures between the fourth ventricle and the subarachnoid space. Such a blockage prevents CSF from leaving the ventricular system, but does not turn off the mechanism that forms CSF. Therefore, CSF continues to be produced and builds up in the system. The ventricles become distended, and the pressure on the brain can destroy its tissue. This condition is called **hydrocephalus**— quite literally, water on (and in) the brain.

Summary

The blood supply to the brain is from the vertebral arteries and the internal carotid arteries. The two vertebral arteries fuse to form the basilar artery. Branches of the vertebral arteries supply the brainstem, cerebellum, and occipital lobes of the cerebrum. The internal carotid arteries branch to form the middle cerebral arteries and the anterior cerebral arteries, which supply the frontal, parietal, and temporal lobes of the cerebrum as well as the diencephalon and deep parts of the cerebrum. The blood-brain barrier limits what molecules are exchanged between the capillaries and brain tissue. Cerebrospinal fluid is a filtrate of blood formed in the brain's ventricles and resorbed back into the bloodstream through specializations in the walls of the venous sinuses of the dura mater.

CHAPTER 3 SUMMARY

The brain is protected by the skull and three meninges (dura mater, arachnoid, and pia mater). Cerebrospinal fluid in the subarachnoid space acts as a shock absorber.

The brain is divisible into the brainstem (medulla, pons, and midbrain), the cerebellum, the diencephalon, and the cerebrum. The ventricular system filled with cerebrospinal fluid, includes the two lateral ventricles of the cerebrum,, the third ventricle of the diencephalon, and the fourth ventricle of the brainstem.

The surface of the brain has many prominent bulges and depressions which are landmarks for underlying nuclei, tracts, and cortical areas with functional significance. Each cerebral hemisphere has four major lobes (frontal, parietal, occipital, and temporal) as well as the insula which is not a part of any of the four lobes.

The brain's blood supply is from the vertebral and internal carotid arteries. Branches of the vertebral arteries supply the brainstem, cerebellum, and occipital lobes of the cerebrum. Branches of the internal carotid arteries supply the frontal, parietal, and temporal lobes of the cerebrum, deep portions of the cerebrum, and the diencephalon. The arterial circle of Willis acts as an anastomotic system interconnecting the vertebral system of arteries with the internal carotid system of arteries. The blood-brain barrier controls what molecules can be exchanged between capillaries and brain tissue. Cerebrospinal fluid is formed in the brain's ventricles and resorbed by specializations in the walls of venous sinuses of the dura mater.

ADDITIONAL READING

Noback, C. R. & Demarest, R. J. (1967). *The human nervous system: Basic principles of neurobiology* (3rd ed.). San Juan, Puerto Rico: McGraw-Hill.

Nolte, J. (1988). *The human brain: An introduction to its functional anatomy* (2nd ed.). St. Louis: C. V. Mosby.

Williams, P. L., Warwick, R., Dyson, M., & Bannister, L. H. (Eds.). (1989). *Gray's anatomy* (37th ed.). Edinburgh: Churchill Livingstone.

STUDY GUIDE

Answer each question with a brief paragraph

1. Describe the structures that protect the brain.
2. Describe the neuraxis.
3. What are the tegmental and nontegmental portions of the brainstem?
4. What are the four divisions of the diencephalon?
5. Describe the ventricular system of the brain.
6. Describe the structure of the midbrain tectum.
7. What is the epithalamus?
8. Describe the two ways of subdividing the cerebellum.
9. Describe the parts of the frontal lobe including gyri and Brodmann's numbers.
10. What is the insula?
11. What parts of the brain are vascularized by the middle cerebral artery?
12. What is the circle of Willis?

Odd One Out

In each of the following questions, choose the item that does not "fit" with the other three; briefly explain what the other three have in common that the odd one lacks. There may be more than one correct answer.

1. ___ braincase

   ___ dura mater

   ___ pia mater

   ___ arachnoid

   WHY?

2. ___ tectum

   ___ pyramids

   ___ olive

   ___ pons proper

   WHY?

3. ___ gracile tubercle

   ___ olive

   ___ lateral lemniscus

   ___ acoustic tubercle

   WHY?

4. ___ Brodmann's area 4

___ Brodmann's areas 3, 1, 2

___ Brodmann's area 17

___ Brodmann's areas 41, 42

WHY?

5. ___ anterior communicating artery

___ posterior communicating artery

___ posterior cerebral artery

___ superior cerebellar artery

WHY?

6. ___ anterior inferior cerebellar artery

___ superior cerebellar artery

___ posterior cerebral artery

___ middle cerebellar artery

WHY?

INTERNAL ORGANIZATION OF THE CENTRAL NERVOUS SYSTEM

Now that you are familiar with the surface anatomy of the brain, it is time to start looking at its internal organization. This will help clarify the relationships of the auditory, speech, language, and vestibular systems to other parts of the central nervous system.

I. NUCLEI AND CORTICES

Specific terms are used for groups of CNS neuronal cell bodies and their dendritic arborizations that have similar morphology and function. Those arranged in clusters are called **nuclei** (singular, **nucleus**; not to be confused with the nuclei of cells); those arranged in layers on the surface of the brain are called **cortices** (singular, **cortex**). Nuclei and cortices together are the **gray matter** of the brain. They are interconnected by the axons of projection neurons, which are the **white matter** (**tracts**) of the CNS.

Although each nucleus and each cortical region has a specific (and often unique) neuronal organization, all CNS gray matter shares some general organizational characteristics. Each nucleus and cortical region contains **local circuit neurons** (**Golgi type II**), which facilitate its information processing. Each also contains **projection neurons** (**Golgi type I**). Their axons form either the tracts that send information to other nuclei or cortical areas, or—in the case of alpha (lower) motor neurons of motor nuclei—the peripheral nerves that innervate skeletal muscles or glands.

This general organizational plan underlies the complex circuitry of the CNS. If you keep this plan in mind, it will provide a framework on which to hang more elaborate schemes.

The organization of the CNS is simplest, and most easily understood, in the spinal cord.

Summary

Nuclei and cortices contain both local circuit neurons and projection neurons. The axons of the projection neurons form the tracts of the central nervous system.

II. SPINAL CORD

Like the brain, the spinal cord is covered by three meninges: dura mater, arachnoid layer, and pia mater. The spinal cord lies completely within the **neural canal** of the vertebral column. However, it is shorter than the vertebral column, extending from the foramen magnum to the lumbar (lower back) region of the vertebral column. Between every pair of vertebrae are holes, the **intervertebral foramina**, through which paired spinal nerves enter and leave the vertebral column. Because the cord is shorter than the column, **spinal nerves** travel for variable distances within the neural canal before exiting.

A. Topography of Spinal Cord

The spinal cord is commonly divided into regions: the **cervical region** in the neck; the **thoracic region** in the chest; the **lumbar region** in the lower back; the **sacral region** in the pelvis; and, below that, the **coccygeal region**, named for the coccyx ("tail bone").

There are 31 pairs of spinal nerves, named for the regions where they enter or leave the vertebral column: 8 pairs of cervical spinal nerves, 12 thoracic, 5 lumbar, 5 sacral, and 1 coccygeal.

The large nerves that innervate the arms and legs enter and leave the spinal cord at swellings, or enlargements, of the cord: the **cervical enlargement** for the arms; the **lumbosacral enlargement** for the legs.

1. Organization of Spinal Nerves

All spinal nerves are similarly organized. They contain both sensory and motor fibers and therefore are called mixed nerves. Sensory and motor fibers, in turn, can be further classified according to the type of information they carry. The terminology can be confusing unless you remember that *a-* is a Latin prefix for *toward* (as in approach) and *-fero* is derived from the Latin word for *to bear or carry*; *afferent* refers to information flowing toward the CNS (i.e., sensory). Similarly, *e-* is a Latin prefix for *away from* (as in exit); *efferent* refers to information *flowing out from* the CNS toward peripheral parts of the body (i.e., motor). The term "general" is used in describing sensory and motor nerve fibers to distinguish them from "special" nerve fibers, which are found in some cranial nerves; more on "special" when we discuss cranial nerves. The types of nerve fibers in spinal nerves are:

- Sensory fibers carrying information from the skin and proprioceptors are **general somatic afferent**, or **GSA**, fibers.
- Sensory fibers carrying information from the viscera (e.g., lungs, digestive tract) are **general visceral afferent**, or **GVA**, fibers.
- Motor fibers innervating the heart, glands, and smooth muscles of viscera and blood vessels are **general visceral efferents**, or **GVE**, fibers.
- Motor fibers innervating skeletal muscles are **general somatic efferent**, or **GSE**, fibers.

Starting at the periphery, each spinal nerve is formed by two contributions: a **dorsal ramus** from the dorsal half of the body and a **ventral ramus** from the ventral half of the body. These rami join just outside the intervertebral foramen to form the **spinal nerve**. The spinal nerve and the two rami that form it all carry both afferent and efferent nerve fibers (GSA and GSE) and so are called mixed nerves (Figure 4–1).

The spinal nerve is then joined by a visceral nerve, called a **ramus communicantis** (plural, rami communicantes), which contains both afferent and efferent visceral nerve fibers (GVA and GVE). Thus when the spinal nerve passes through the intervertebral foramen into the vertebral column it contains all four types of nerve fibers (GSA, GVA, GVE, and GSE) (Figure 4–1).

Inside the vertebral column, the spinal nerve divides into a **dorsal root** and a **ventral root**. The dorsal root is entirely sensory, containing only GSA and GVA fibers. It also contains the cell bodies of the unipolar sensory neurons—both GVA and GSA—that form the **dorsal root ganglion**. The central fibers of these unipolar neurons continue in the dorsal root and enter the dorsolateral aspect of the spinal cord.

The ventral root is entirely motor, containing only GVE and GSE fibers. Its fibers exit ventrolaterally from the spinal cord (Figure 4–1).

To summarize, sensory information travels from the dorsal and ventral rami and rami communicantes to the spinal nerve. It enters the cord dorsolaterally, in the dorsal root of the spinal nerve (which contains the dorsal root ganglion). Motor information leaves the cord ventrolaterally in the ventral root, which then joins the spinal nerve. From the spinal nerve, motor information travels to effector organs (muscles and glands) via the dorsal and ventral rami and rami communicantes.

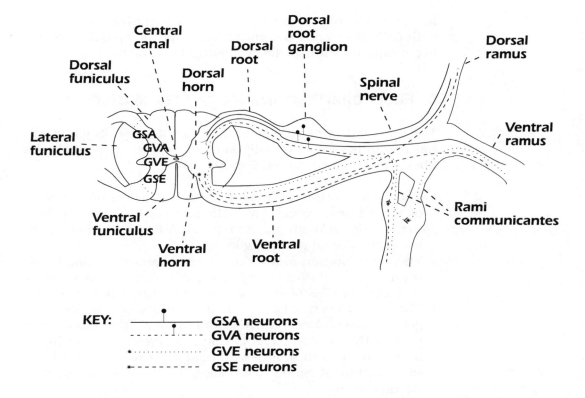

Figure 4–1. A diagrammatic cross-section of the spinal cord and one spinal nerve showing the organization of spinal nerves. Only a very few of the hundreds to thousands of neurons in a spinal nerve are shown. GSA = general somatic afferent; GSE = general somatic efferent; GVA = general visceral afferent; GVE = general visceral efferent.

B. Internal Organization of Spinal Cord

White matter forms the outer portion of the cord; gray matter forms the inner, deeper portions. The white matter is divided into large groups of tracts called **funiculi**: there are a **dorsal**, two **lateral**, and a **ventral** funiculus, named for the portion of the cord they occupy (Figure 4–1). These funiculi contain all the tracts of the spinal cord.

When the cord is cut in cross-section, the gray matter has the shape of a butterfly with spread wings. The upper parts of the two "wings" are the **dorsal horns**; the lower portions, the **ventral horns**. In the thoracic and sacral portions of the cord, where there are many general visceral efferent (GVE) neurons, there is also a small **lateral horn** between the dorsal and ventral horns (Figure 4–1).

In the very center of the cord is a small **central canal** filled with CSF. It extends the entire length of the spinal cord and is continuous with the fourth ventricle of the medulla.

C. Functional Organization of Gray Matter

The gray matter of the spinal cord is organized in longitudinal columns of functionally similar neurons, in which the fiber types are segregated (Figure 4–1).

- The upper portion of the dorsal horn consists of a column of second order general somatic afferent (GSA) cell bodies. Synapsing on them are primary GSA fibers from cell bodies in the dorsal root ganglia.
- The lower portion of the dorsal horn contains a small column of general visceral afferent (GVA) neurons. Synapsing on them are GVA fibers from dorsal root ganglion neurons.
- The lateral horn, when present, consists of cell bodies of general visceral efferent (GVE) neurons. Their axons form part of the ventral roots of spinal nerves that eventually innervate smooth muscles and glands (see the box "Motor Innervation of Smooth Muscles, Cardiac Muscles, and Glands" below).
- The ventral horn consists of a large column of cell bodies of **alpha motor neurons** (GSE) whose axons enter the ventral roots of spinal nerves and innervate skeletal muscles and of smaller **gamma motor neurons** whose axons innervate the intrafusal muscle cells of muscle spindles (see Chapter 2 box on Muscle Spindles).

D. Functional Organization of White Matter

The white matter of the cord is also precisely organized. It is made up of the axons of projection neurons from cell bodies in dorsal root ganglia, spinal cord gray matter, and neural centers in the brain.

Remember that tracts are always composed of the axons of projection neurons.

The tracts that form the white matter immediately surrounding the gray matter of the cord are collectively called **fasciculi proprii**. They connect one part of the spinal cord with another and are important in reflexes.

The rest of the white matter of the spinal cord is divided into the major sensory tracts, which carry information from the spinal cord up to the brain, and the major motor tracts,

MOTOR INNERVATION OF SMOOTH MUSCLES, CARDIAC MUSCLES, AND GLANDS

The motor innervation of smooth muscles, cardiac muscles, and glands (GVE) is distinctly different from the motor innervation of skeletal muscles (GSE).

- Contraction of skeletal muscles is almost always under volitional control; contraction of smooth and cardiac muscles, and secretions of glands, are almost entirely involuntary.
- All GSE fibers are excitatory—causing contraction of skeletal muscle cells. Some GVE fibers are excitatory but others are inhibitory (i.e., some cause muscle contraction or secretions whereas others inhibit muscle contractions or secretions).

Together the GVE neurons make up the autonomic nervous system, which controls involuntary or "autonomous" excitation or inhibition. The autonomic nervous system is divided into a sympathetic system, arising from the thoracic and lumbar regions of the spinal cord, and a parasympathetic system, arising from the brainstem and sacral region of the spinal cord.

- Sympathetic fibers course in thoracic and lumbar spinal nerves; they prepare the body for emergency situations by causing events like increased heart rate and blood pressure.
- Parasympathetic fibers course in the sacral spinal nerves and cranial nerves and decrease heart rate and blood pressure, thus putting the body in a state that facilitates calm, easy-going behavior and good digestion.

The central control of both the sympathetic and parasympathetic systems lies in the hypothalamus. Their peripheral portions consist of two-neuron chains. The first neuron has its cell body in the CNS (brainstem or spinal cord); its axon enters the PNS and then synapses with neurons whose cell bodies comprise peripheral autonomic ganglia. The axons of these autonomic ganglion cells then synapse with smooth muscle cells, cardiac muscle cells, or gland cells.

For the sake of simplicity, this text does not include the autonomic ganglia of cranial nerves with GVE fibers. However, note that all GVE fibers do synapse with autonomic ganglion cells whose axons then innervate the effector cells.

---

which carry information from the brain down to the gray matter of the spinal cord.

1. Major Sensory Tracts

The largest and functionally most significant of the sensory (afferent) tracts carrying information from the cord to the brain are the **dorsal columns**, the **spinothalamic tract**, and the **spinocerebellar tracts** (Figure 4–2).

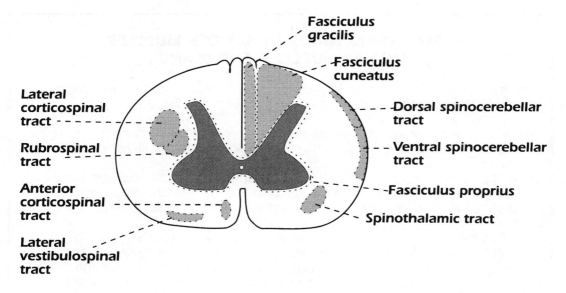

Figure 4–2. Diagram of a cross-section of the cervical spinal cord showing the position of the major sensory tracts on the right and the major motor tracts on the left. Fasciculi proprii are shown on both sides. The gray matter is the central dark stipple.

a. Dorsal Columns The dorsal columns, which make up the bulk of the dorsal funiculus, are formed by the central processes of dorsal root ganglion cells. They carry information about fine (discriminative) touch, pressure, and proprioception to the brainstem. There are two dorsal columns, called fasciculi (singular, fasciculus) on each side. The **fasciculus gracilis**, which lies medially, carries lower body information (from approximately the waist down). The **fasciculus cuneatus**, which lies laterally, carries upper body information (from approximately the waist up to the back of the head).

This information is processed in the brainstem and transmitted to a thalamic nucleus, where it is further processed before being transmitted to the somesthetic portion of the cerebral cortex (areas 3, 1, and 2).

b. Spinothalamic Tract The spinothalamic tract lies partially in the lateral and partially in the ventral funiculus. Its cell bodies are in the dorsal horns of the gray matter of the opposite side. These tracts ascend through the cord and brainstem, synapse with thalamic nuclei, and finally project to the somesthetic cortex (areas 3, 1, and 2). The spinothalamic system carries information about pain, temperature, and gross touch (as opposed to discriminative touch).

c. Spinocerebellar Tracts There are two right-left pairs of spinocerebellar tracts: the **dorsal spinocerebellar tract**, forming the dorsal surface of the lateral funiculus, and the **ventral spinocerebellar tract**, forming the ventral surface of the lateral funiculus. These tracts carry primarily proprioceptive information from the gray matter of the spinal cord up to the cerebellum.

2. Major Motor Tracts

Major motor (efferent) tracts carry information from the brain to the alpha (lower) and gamma (also lower) motor neurons, which lie in the ventral horns of the spinal cord. Those to which we'll refer in later chapters are the **lateral** and **anterior corticospinal tracts**, the **rubrospinal tract**, and the **lateral vestibulospinal tract** (Figure 4–2).

a. Lateral Corticospinal Tract The largest efferent tract is the lateral corticospinal tract, which runs in the lateral funiculus. Its cell bodies lie within the cerebral cortex on the opposite side. Its axons, after leaving the cerebral cortex via the internal capsule, travel in the cerebral peduncles and then through the ventral pons as **corticospinal fibers**. When they emerge from the ventral pons, these corticospinal fibers form the **pyramids** of the lower medulla. They then cross in the **pyramidal decussation** to form the lateral corticospinal tract, which finally terminates on the alpha (lower) motor neurons in the ventral horns of the spinal cord gray matter.

Actually there are usually small local circuit neurons that receive the information, and their axons synapse with the lower motor neurons. This is true for all the tracts to lower motor neurons.

b. Anterior Corticospinal Tract Some corticospinal fibers, instead of crossing in the pyramidal decussation, enter the spinal cord on the same side. They form the anterior corticospinal tract, which travels in the ventral funiculus and crosses the midline shortly before synapsing on cells of the ventral horn of the spinal cord.

Both the lateral and anterior corticospinal fibers control primarily those lower motor neurons that innervate extensor muscles.

c. Rubrospinal Tract The rubrospinal tract, like the lateral corticospinal tract, lies in the lateral funiculus. It primarily controls the lower motor neurons that go to the flexor muscles of the extremities. Its cell bodies are located in the red nucleus of the midbrain tegmentum on the opposite side. After crossing the midline, its axons pass through the lower portion of the brainstem to form the rubrospinal tracts. Eventually they terminate in the ventral horn of the spinal cord.

d. Lateral Vestibulospinal Tract The cell bodies of the lateral vestibulospinal tract are located in the vestibular nuclei of the medulla. Their axons travel down the spinal cord in the ventral funiculus and terminate on lower motor neurons that innervate extensor muscles of the extremities.

Summary

Spinal nerves are formed by the convergence of nerve fibers of the dorsal rami, ventral rami, and rami communicantes. Motor fibers (GSE and GVE) are in the ventral roots; sensory fibers (GSA and GVA) are in the dorsal roots. All the cell bodies of sensory fibers are in the dorsal root ganglia.

The white matter of the spinal cord forms the two lateral funiculi, the dorsal funiculus, and the ventral funiculus. They contain the sensory and motor tracts of the spinal cord. The sensory tracts are dorsal columns, spinothalamic tract, and spinocerebellar tracts; the motor tracts are lateral and anterior corticospinal tracts, rubrospinal tract, and lateral vestibulospinal tract.

The gray matter of the spinal cord contains the dorsal horn (GSA and GVA), the lateral horn (GVE), and the anterior horn (GSE).

III. INTERNAL ORGANIZATION OF BRAINSTEM

Because of the diverse functions of the brainstem, the "variations on the theme" are much more complex than the "theme" of the spinal cord.

The pattern of organization established in the spinal cord continues into the tegmentum of the brainstem—the medulla, pontine tegmentum, and midbrain tegmentum. There it becomes a theme with variations. The paired spinal nerves, which exit the vertebral column between every pair of vertebrae, are replaced by paired **cranial nerves**, which are less regularly arranged and more diverse in their structure. The columns of continuous spinal cord gray matter give way to discontinuous brainstem nuclei—at least one for each cranial nerve. The brainstem also includes many tracts that carry information to and from the spinal cord, and other tracts and nuclei that are not directly related to cranial nerves.

A. Cranial Nerves and Their Nuclei

There are 12 cranial nerves; they are designated by Roman numerals. Cranial nerve I (the **olfactory nerve**) attaches to the **olfactory bulb** of the cerebrum and cranial nerve II (the **optic nerve**) to the diencephalon; they were described in Chapter 3. Cranial nerves III through XII attach directly to the brainstem (Table 4–1).

Many cranial nerves contain "special" as well as "general" nerve fibers. In sensory (afferent) nerves, the "special" fibers are those from the special senses (smell, vision, taste, hearing, and balance). In motor (efferent) nerves, the "special" fibers are those innervating skeletal muscles of visceral (embryological) origin. These visceral muscles are "special" in that they are striated and under voluntary control, as opposed to smooth visceral muscles, which are *not* striated and *not* under voluntary control.

The brainstem cranial nerves can be classified according to the fibers they carry.

- *Cranial nerves III, IV, VI, and XII (oculomotor, trochlear, abducens, and hypoglossal)* are composed primarily or entirely of axons innervating general somatic skeletal muscles; they are GSE nerves.
- *Cranial nerve VIII (vestibulocochlear)* contains only nerve fibers for the special senses of hearing and equilibrium; it is a special somatic afferent nerve (SSA) carrying only SSA fibers—as opposed to general somatic afferent fibers (GSA), which carry sensation from general senses such as touch, pressure, and proprioception.
- *Cranial nerves V, VII, IX, X, and XI (trigeminal, facial, glossopharyngeal, vagus, and spinal accessory)* contain at least some axons that innervate special visceral muscles and are thus special visceral efferent fibers (SVE). Special visceral muscles develop from the walls of the upper respiratory and upper digestive tracts. Unlike other visceral muscles they are striated and under voluntary control. All these nerves except XI (spinal accessory) also have sensory fibers and thus are mixed nerves.

1. Nerves with GSE Fibers

Cranial nerves III, IV, VI, and XII are the only cranial nerves with general somatic efferent (GSE) axons. Their nuclei are

Table 4–1
Components of cranial nerves.

Cranial Nerve	Fiber Types	Ganglia	Central Connections
I Olfactory (smell)	SVA	—	Olfactory bulb
II Optic (vision)	SSA	In retina	Lateral geniculate body
III Oculomotor	GSE	—	Oculomotor nucleus
	GVE	—	Edinger-Westphal nucleus
IV Trochlear	GSE	—	Trochlear nucleus
V Trigeminal	GSA	Trigeminal	Chief nucleus of V
	GSA	Trigeminal	Descending nucleus of V
	GSA	—	Mesencephalic nucleus of V
	SVE	—	Masticator nucleus
VI Abducens	GSE	—	Abducens nucleus
VII Facial	GSA	Geniculate	Descending nucleus of V
	SVA	Geniculate	Nucleus solitarius (taste)
	GVE	—	Superior salivatory nucleus
	SVE	—	Facial nucleus
VIII Vestibulocochlear	SSA	Spiral	Cochlear nuclei (hearing)
	SSA	Vestibular	Vestibular nuclei
IX Glossopharyngeal	GSA	Inferior glossopharynegeal	Descending nucleus of V
	SVA	Superior glossopharyngeal	Nucleus solitarius (taste)
	GVA	Inferior glossopharyngeal	Nucleus solitarius (nontaste)
	GVE	—	Inferior salivatory nucleus
	SVE	—	Nucleus ambiguus
X Vagus	GSA	Superior vagal	Descending nucleus of V
	SVA	Inferior vagal	Nucleus solitarius (taste)
	GVA	Inferior vagal	Nucleus solitarius (nontaste)
	GVE	—	Dorsal motor nucleus of X
	SVE	—	Nucleus ambiguus
XI Spinal accessory	SVE (cranial)	—	Nucleus ambiguus

Table 4–1 (continued)

Cranial Nerve	Fiber Types	Ganglia	Central Connections
	SVE (spinal)	—	Accessory nucleus
XII Hypoglossal	GSE	—	Hypoglossal nucleus

comparable to the ventral horn column of the spinal cord. However, because not all cranial nerves contain GSE fibers, these brainstem nuclei are discontinuous, rather than forming a continuous column as their counterparts do in the cord (Figure 4–3).

a. Oculomotor Nerve (Cranial Nerve III) This nerve innervates four of the six somatic motor muscles that attach the eyeball to the bony orbit and cause eye movements; they are collectively called the **extrinsic ocular muscles** (as opposed to intrinsic ocular muscles, which are located within the eyeball). The cell bodies of these nerve fibers form the **oculomotor nucleus**, which lies in the midbrain tegmentum just below and lateral to the cerebral aqueduct. The fibers from this nucleus travel ventrally and leave the brainstem from the **interpeduncular fossa** (Figure 4–3).

The oculomotor nerve also has a small general visceral efferent (GVE) nucleus, the **Edinger-Westphal nucleus**, which lies adjacent to the oculomotor nucleus (Figure 4–3). Its axons go out to the smooth muscles that focus the eye and control the size of the pupil.

b. Trochlear Nerve (Cranial Nerve IV) The trochlear nerve contains only general somatic efferent (GSE) fibers that extend out to a single extrinsic ocular muscle. Its cell bodies form the **trochlear nucleus** (GSE), which lies just below the cerebral aqueduct at the border between midbrain and pons. The axons from the trochlear nucleus pass dorsally, cross the midline above the cerebral aqueduct, and leave the brain dorsally at the junction between pons and midbrain (Figure 4–3). This is the only cranial nerve that exits the brain dorsally and the only one whose axons decussate.

c. Abducens Nerve (Cranial Nerve VI) The abducens nerve also contains only GSE fibers; they go to the remaining extrinsic ocular muscle. The abducens nucleus lies just under the fourth ventricle in the lower pontine tegmentum (Figure

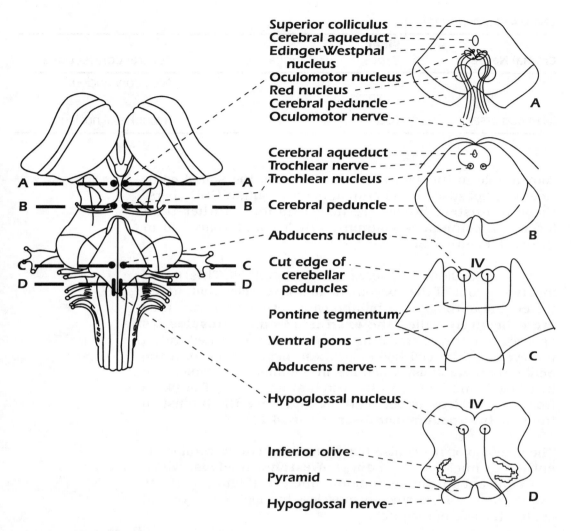

Superior colliculus
Cerebral aqueduct
Edinger-Westphal nucleus
Oculomotor nucleus
Red nucleus
Cerebral peduncle
Oculomotor nerve

A

Cerebral aqueduct
Trochlear nerve
Trochlear nucleus

Cerebral peduncle

B

Abducens nucleus

Cut edge of cerebellar peduncles

IV

Pontine tegmentum

Ventral pons

Abducens nerve

C

Hypoglossal nucleus

IV

Inferior olive

Pyramid

Hypoglossal nerve

D

Figure 4–3. Dorsal view of the brainstem and diencephalon (left side of figure) showing the locations of the oculomotor, trochlear, abducens, and hypoglossal nuclei. **A**, **B**, **C**, and **D** are cross-sections of the brainstem at indicated locations showing the positions of the nuclei and exiting cranial nerves. IV = fourth ventricle.

4–3). Its fibers pass ventrally to exit the brain just lateral to the pyramid at the junction of the medulla and pons.

d. Hypoglossal Nerve (Cranial Nerve XII) The hypoglossal nerve innervates both the intrinsic and extrinsic musculature of the tongue. The lower (alpha and gamma) motor neurons (GSE) that form the **hypoglossal nucleus** lie in the medulla, just under the fourth ventricle on either side of the midline; their axons pass ventrally from the hypoglossal nucleus to exit the brain in the groove between the pyramid and the olive (Figure 4–3).

2. Special Sensory Nerve: Vestibulocochlear Nerve (cranial nerve VIII)

This brainstem cranial nerve contains only special somatic afferents (SSA)—called special rather than general because they carry the sensory information of two special senses, hearing and balance. Their cell bodies are bipolar neurons.

a. Cochlear Division The bipolar neurons for hearing form the **spiral ganglion** in the cochlea. Their peripheral processes go out to the sensory cells for hearing. Their central processes form the **cochlear division** of the **vestibulocochlear nerve**, enter the brainstem at the cerebellopontine angle, and terminate in the **cochlear nuclear complex** at the junction of the pons and medulla (Figure 4–4). We will have more details about the cochlear nuclei when we discuss the auditory pathways in Chapter 7.

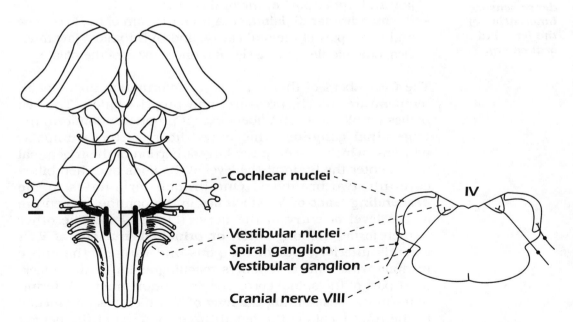

Figure 4–4. Dorsal view of brainstem and diencephalon (left side of figure) showing the locations of the cochlear and vestibular nuclei. Right side of figure is a cross-section at the indicated location showing the position of these nuclei and the entering vestibulocochlear (VIII) cranial nerve. IV = fourth ventricle.

b. Vestibular Division The bipolar neurons for balance form the **vestibular ganglion**, also called **Scarpa's ganglion**. Their peripheral processes go out to the sensory cells of the **vestibular apparatus**. Their central processes enter the brainstem adjacent to the cochlear division at the cerebellopontine angle and project to the **vestibular nuclei**, a group of nuclei lying just deep to the floor of the fourth ventricle (Figure 4–4). More details will be found in Chapter 5, on the vestibular system.

3. Nerves with SVE Fibers

Cranial nerves V, VII, IX, X, and XI contain SVE fibers innervating special visceral muscles.

a. Trigeminal Nerve (Cranial Nerve V) The **trigeminal nerve** (tri = three; gem = part) has three major divisions, only one of which contains SVE fibers:

This is the largest of the 12 cranial nerves; its size reflects the dense sensory innervation of the face and oral cavity.

- the **ophthalmic division**, GSA from the skin of the upper part of the face including the region around the nose, eye, and forehead;
- the **maxillary division**, GSA from the skin of the upper jaw and upper part of the oral cavity;
- the **mandibular division**, GSA from the skin of the lower jaw and lower part of the oral cavity; and SVE to most jaw muscles, one middle ear muscle, and one muscle of the palate.

The GSA fibers of this nerve carry information about pain, temperature, touch, pressure, and proprioception. The cell bodies for all these GSA fibers except proprioception form the **trigeminal ganglion**. The central fibers of these unipolar neurons, which make up the largest portion of the trigeminal nerve, enter the brain at the level of the pons and then bifurcate into two branches. One branch terminates in the **descending tract of V**, which lies in the pontine tegmentum at the level of entry of the nerve (Figure 4–5). The other branch forms the long **chief, or principal, nucleus of V**. It extends inferiorly out of the pons and through the entire medulla with some of its fibers reaching as far as the uppermost part of the spinal cord. The descending tract of V terminates in the **descending nucleus of V**, which lies just medial to the tract for its entire length from the level of the nerve's entry into the brainstem all the way to the uppermost part of the spinal cord (Figure 4–5).

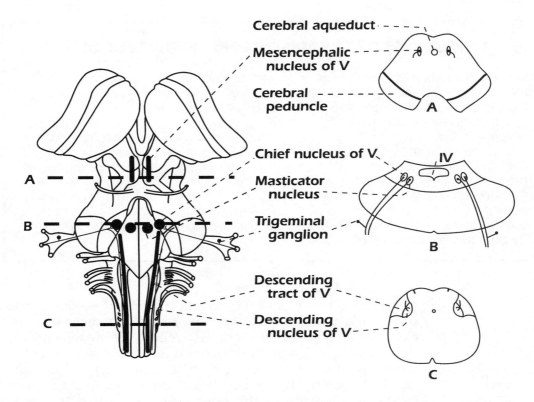

Figure 4–5. Dorsal view of brainstem and and diencephalon (left side of figure) showing the locations of the trigeminal nuclei and ganglion. **A**, **B**, and **C** are cross-sections of the brainstem at indicated locations showing the positions of the nuclei, tracts, and nerve. IV = fourth ventricle.

Both the chief nucleus of V and the descending nucleus of V are made up of second order somesthetic neurons of the trigeminal system. Their large size reflects the dense innervation of the skin of the face and oral cavity.

The cell bodies of the proprioceptive neurons in the trigeminal nerve lie in the midbrain and form the **mesencephalic nucleus of V**. Their peripheral fibers come from muscle spindles, Golgi tendon organs, and joint receptors including those of the temporomandibular joint. The central fibers of those unipolar neurons terminate on neurons of the chief nucleus of V and descending nucleus of V. They also send collaterals to the **motor nucleus of V**. (See the box, "Uniqueness of the Mesencephalic Nucleus of V.")

The mesencephalic nucleus of V is the only place where cell bodies of primary sensory neurons are in the CNS rather than in a peripheral ganglion.

<hr>

UNIQUENESS OF THE MESENCEPHALIC NUCLEUS OF V

With one exception, the cell bodies of primary sensory neurons are in ganglia of the PNS, either dorsal root ganglia of spinal nerves or sensory ganglia of cranial nerves. The exception is the primary proprioceptive neurons of the trigeminal nerve.

These neurons, like most primary sensory neurons, are unipolar. However, their peripheral fibers enter the CNS and their cell bodies are in the mesencephalic nucleus of V in the midbrain. Their central fibers are wholly within the CNS; they synapse with both the lower motor neurons of the masticator nucleus and the sensory neurons of the thalamus (VPM; described in Section II D of this chapter).

Developmental studies have shown that the neurons of the mesencephalic nucleus of V first develop outside of the developing brain and then migrate into the brain as development continues. Neither the evolutionary nor the functional reasons for this unusual migration are understood.

<hr>

"Masticator" refers to chewing, as in mastication.

All the SVE neurons of the central trigeminal system are in the mandibular division. They innervate the major jaw muscles (muscles of mastication), as well as the mylohyoideus, the anterior belly of the digastricus, the tensor tympani muscle of the middle ear, and the tensor veli palatini muscle of the palate. The cell bodies of these motor neurons lie in the tegmentum of the pons, just medial to the chief nucleus of V, and form the **motor nucleus of V** (also called the **masticator nucleus**); the axons pass out through the pons as the motor root of the trigeminal nerve and leave the pons adjacent to the sensory root of the fifth cranial nerve.

b. Facial Nerve (Cranial Nerve VII) The **facial nerve** has two sensory and two motor components.

- A small GSA component innervates part of the skin of the external ear.
- SVA fibers carry information from the taste buds on the anterior two-thirds of the tongue.
- A large SVE component innervates primarily the muscles of facial expression, or mimetic muscles (from Greek word for actor; mime and mimic come from the same root). Other SVE fibers innervate the stylohyoideus, the posterior belly of the digastricus, and the stapedius muscle of the middle ear.
- GVE fibers innervate the lacrimal (tear) gland and two salivary glands of the head, the submandibular and sublingual glands.

The cell bodies for both types of sensory (afferent) fibers of the facial nerve are unipolar cells in the **geniculate gan-**

glion. It lies in the temporal bone, in the bony canal that carries the facial nerve.

- The GSA central fibers of geniculate ganglion cells enter the brainstem with the rest of the facial nerve adjacent to cranial nerve VIII, and then go to a small portion of the **descending nucleus of V**—which, as we have seen, is the largest GSA nucleus for sensory information from the face (Figure 4–6).
- The SVA fibers of taste separate from the GSA fibers within the pontine tegmentum and synapse there on neurons of the gustatory (taste) portion of the **nucleus solitarius**.

The motor portions, both SVE and GVE, of the facial nerve have their own nuclei of origin in the medulla.

- The SVE nucleus is the **facial nucleus**, a large nucleus located in the pontine tegmentum. Instead of leaving the brainstem directly, its axons travel to the floor of the fourth ventricle, wrap around the abducens nucleus, move out ventrally and laterally, and leave the brain with the rest of the facial nerve. They go to the muscles of facial expression and a few other muscles including the stapedius.
- The GVE component is small. Its nucleus, the **superior salivatory nucleus** in the upper medulla (Figure 4–6), sends information out to the sublingual and submandibular salivary glands and the lacrimal (tear) gland.

c. Glossopharyngeal Nerve (Cranial Nerve IX) The organization of the **glossopharyngeal nerve** is similar to that of the facial nerve. It includes the same four fiber types plus GVA fibers (Figure 4–7):

- a small GSA component from the external ear;
- an SVA component carrying taste information from the posterior one-third of the tongue;
- a GVA component carrying information from the mucosa of the Eustachian tube and the upper pharynx;
- an SVE component going to the stylopharyngeus muscle; and
- a GVE component to the parotid salivary gland.

The three sensory components of the glossopharyngeal nerve have unipolar cell bodies that lie just outside the brainstem in a pair of ganglia called the **superior** and **inferior ganglia of the glossopharyngeal nerve**. The central processes of these neurons segregate into functional groups as they enter the CNS in the groove just dorsal to the olive and go to their destinations (Figure 4–7):

The facial nerve is the only cranial nerve that travels through a long bony tunnel, rather than a foramen, as it leaves the braincase. Because of this trajectory, the nerve may be compressed along the way. This explains why facial nerve palsies are more common than palsies in other cranial nerves.

The nucleus solitarius has both a taste (gustatory) portion and a nontaste portion for general visceral afferents.

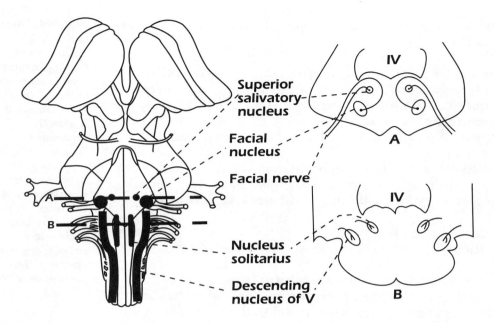

Figure 4–6. Dorsal view of brainstem and diencephalon (left side of figure) showing the locations of the nuclei of the facial nerve. **A** and **B** are cross-sections of the brainstem at indicated locations showing the positions of the nuclei and nerve root. IV = fourth ventricle.

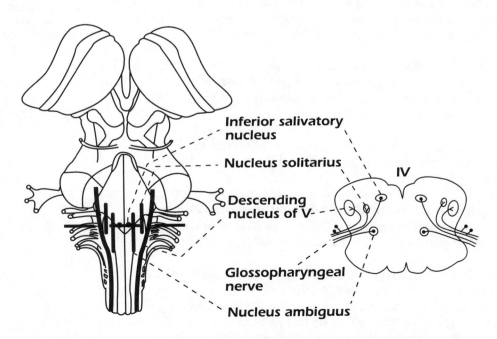

Figure 4–7. Dorsal view of brainstem and diencephalon (left side of figure) showing the locations of the nuclei of the glossopharyngeal nerve. Right side of figure is a cross-section at the indicated location showing the position of the nuclei and the glossopharyngeal nerve. IV = fourth ventricle.

- GSA fibers to the **descending nucleus of V**;
- SVA fibers to the gustatory portion of the **solitarius nucleus**; and
- GVA fibers to the nongustatory portion of the **nucleus solitarius**.

The motor components of the glossopharyngeal nerve are small.

- SVE cell bodies make up the rostral-most portion of a long medullary SVE nucleus, the **nucleus ambiguus**. The lower (alpha and gamma) motor neurons that innervate the stylopharyngeus muscle arise here and pass out of the brain with the rest of the glossopharyngeal nerve in the groove just above the olive.
- GVE cell bodies are in a small medullary nucleus called the **inferior salivatory nucleus**; their axons innervate the secretory cells of the parotid salivary gland.

Note: there is no "o" in "ambiguus."

   d. Vagus Nerve (Cranial Nerve X) The **vagus nerve** (whose name comes from the same root as vagabond, one who wanders) is also called the wandering nerve. It does just that through the neck, thorax, and a large portion of the abdomen.

Many students tend to spell this nerve as vegas. It has nothing to do with Las Vegas. It does relate to vagabond.

The vagus nerve has the same five types of fibers as does the glossopharyngeal nerve (Figure 4–8):

- a small GSA component from a part of the external ear;
- a very small SVA component from taste buds on and near the epiglottis;
- a large GVA component carrying sensory information from the major viscera of the abdomen and thorax, and from the mucosal linings of the larynx and lower pharynx;
- an SVE component that innervates most of the palatal and pharyngeal muscles; and
- a large GVE component that innervates the glands, cardiac muscles, and smooth muscles of thoracic and abdominal organs (heart, lungs, stomach, small intestines).

The cell bodies for the sensory components of the vagus nerve are unipolar; they comprise the **superior** and **inferior ganglia of the vagus nerve**, which lie just outside the medulla of the brainstem. Their central processes enter the brainstem (Figure 4–8) and segregate into:

- a GSA component to the **descending nucleus of V**;
- an SVA component to the gustatory portion of the **nucleus solitarius**; and
- a GVA component to the non-gustatory portion of the **nucleus solitarius**.

The gustatory part of nucleus solitarius receives from cranial nerves VII, IX, and X.

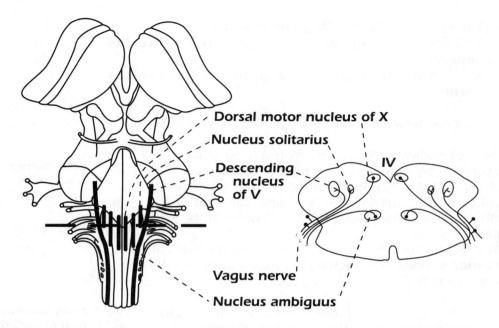

Figure 4–8. Dorsal view of brainstem and diencephalon (left side of figure) showing the locations of the nuclei of the vagus nerve. Right side of figure is a cross-section at the indicated level showing the position of the nuclei and vagus nerve. IV = fourth ventricle.

On the motor side:

- Cell bodies of SVE fibers make up the bulk of the **nucleus ambiguus** in the medulla; the axons exit the brain in the groove just above the olive and innervate most of the palatal and pharyngeal muscles.
- GVE cell bodies are in their own nucleus, the **dorsal motor nucleus of X**, which lies just below the fourth ventricle lateral to the general somatic efferent column. Its axons exit from the groove just above the olive and descend with other vagus nerve fibers to smooth muscle and gland cells of the viscera of the thorax and abdomen, and to cardiac muscle cells of the heart.

    e. Spinal Accessory Nerve (Cranial Nerve XI) The **spinal accessory nerve**, which has only SVE fibers, is divided into a cranial and a spinal portion (Figure 4–9).

Note that axons from nucleus ambiguus contribute to parts of cranial nerves IX, X, and XI.

- The **cranial portion** arises in the medulla from cell bodies in the inferior portion of the nucleus ambiguus. Their axons leave the brain in the groove just above the olive, join the vagus nerve, then separate from the vagus nerve

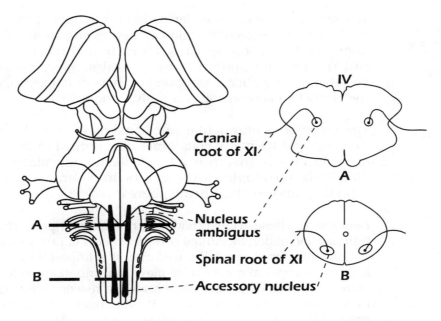

Figure 4–9. Dorsal view of brainstem and diencephalon (left side of figure) showing the location of the nuclei of the spinal accessory nerves. **A** and **B** are cross-sections at the indicated levels showing the position of the spinal accessory nuclei and nerve roots. IV = fourth ventricle.

as the superior laryngeal and recurrent laryngeal nerves to innervate the intrinsic muscles of the larynx.

- The **spinal portion** arises from the cell bodies in the **accessory nucleus** located in the uppermost part of the spinal cord (Figure 4–9). Their axons leave the spinal cord laterally, pass up through the foramen magnum into the cranial cavity, briefly join the cranial portion of the spinal accessory nerve, and then go out to innervate two muscles: the sternocleidomastoideus, a large muscle of the neck, and the upper portion of the trapezius, a large muscle of the back.

B. Reticular Formation

So far we have discussed discrete brainstem structures with specific sensory or motor functions. The brainstem also contains nuclei and their axons whose structures are diffuse and whose functions are nonspecific. Collectively, these elements are called the **reticular formation**.

The reticular formation also contains respiratory centers.

The nuclei of the reticular formation are scattered throughout the brainstem tegmental regions. They receive axon collaterals from specific sensory systems; an individual reticular neuron can receive information from several sensory modalities. Together, they gather information on how much sensory input the brainstem is receiving at any given moment.

The projections of reticular nuclei axons are equally diffuse. An axon and its many collaterals may spread to large areas of the brain—for instance, a single axon and collaterals may distribute terminals to the cerebellum, brainstem, diencephalon, and cerebral hemispheres.

Because of these widespread but nonspecific properties, the reticular formation facilitates several aspects of our lives that we usually take for granted. For instance, it is important in controlling our sleep-wake cycles. It plays an important role in our state of consciousness, whether we are asleep, alert, drowsy, hyperexcited, or even comatose. It has important inputs to the respiratory centers that control respiratory rhythm.

The reticular formation is complex. For our purposes, however, it is enough to consider it as a general, nonspecific portion of the CNS that responds to incoming information by affecting the general state of consciousness and alertness.

C. Two Other Prominent Nuclei of the Tegmental Region of the Brainstem

Two other brainstem nuclei play roles in speech mechanisms.

1. Inferior Olivary Nucleus

You may have heard of olivary nuclei in the auditory pathways. These are superior olivary nuclei and have nothing to do with the inferior olivary nucleus.

The first is the **inferior olivary nucleus**, which is seen as a bulge, called the **olive**, on the ventrolateral aspect of the medulla (Figure 4–3D). This very large nucleus receives information from axons of cells in the cerebral cortex, processes it, and then transmits the processed information to the cerebellum. The **olivocerebellar axons** carrying that information cross the midline and then form a large part of the **restiform body** before entering the cerebellum.

2. Red Nucleus

The largest nucleus of the midbrain tegmentum is the **red nucleus**. It lies next to the midline in the central portion of the midbrain tegmentum (Figure 4–3A). It receives massive axonal input from the cerebral cortex. Its axons in turn give rise to the rubrospinal tracts; they cross the midline in the midbrain tegmentum, descend through the rest of the brainstem tegmentum, continue as the **rubrospinal tracts** in the lateral funiculus of the spinal cord, and finally synapse on ventral horn cells.

D. Somesthetic Pathways of the Brainstem

In discussing the spinal cord we followed the somesthetic senses of discriminative touch, pressure, and proprioception in the **fasciculus gracilis** and **fasciculus cuneatus**. These dorsal column tracts continue into the brainstem as far as the lower edge of the fourth ventricle (its obex). There they terminate in the **gracile** and **cuneate nuclei** (Figure 4–10), which are marked externally by swellings called the **gracile** and **cuneate tubercles**. The cell bodies of these nuclei process the discriminative touch, pressure, and proprioception information. Their axons leave the gracile and cuneate nuclei, and then change both their names and their directions: as the **internal arcuate fibers** they swing ventrally and cross the midline; then, as the **medial lemniscus**, they turn and move rostrally to the **thalamus** (Figure 4–10). These axons end in the **ventral posterior lateral nucleus of the thalamus**, abbreviated **VPL**.

Before finishing this chapter, you will learn about several other thalamic nuclei.

Somesthetic information of pain, temperature, and crude touch is carried by **spinothalamic tracts** from the spinal cord. They pass through the entire brainstem and then also synapse on cells in the **VPL** of the thalamus.

Somesthetic sensations on the face and oral cavity stimulate primary GSA neurons of the trigeminal nerve (and small components of the facial, glossopharyngeal, and vagus nerves that carry somesthetic information from the skin of the external ear). You will recall that these trigeminal GSA fibers terminate on the **chief nucleus of V** and **descending nucleus of V**, whose neurons are the second order somesthetic cells of the facial representation of somesthetic senses (Figure 4–10).

Most axons from the chief and descending nuclei of V swing across the midline in the brainstem and then, as the **ventral trigeminothalamic tract**, ascend to the **ventral posterior medial nucleus of the thalamus**, or **VPM**, which lies just medial to VPL. Some axons do not cross the midline; they form the **dorsal trigeminothalamic tract** to **VPM** on the same side.

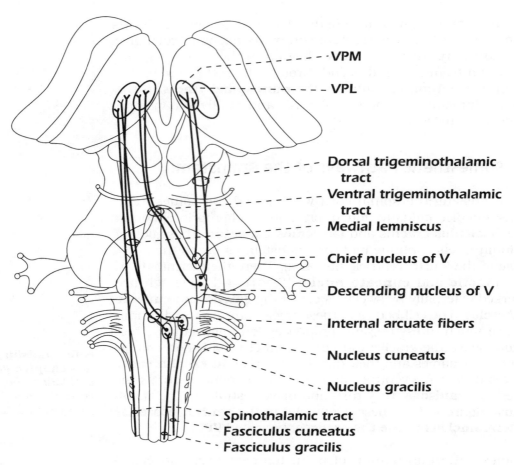

VPM

VPL

Dorsal trigeminothalamic tract

Ventral trigeminothalamic tract

Medial lemniscus

Chief nucleus of V

Descending nucleus of V

Internal arcuate fibers

Nucleus cuneatus

Nucleus gracilis

Spinothalamic tract
Fasciculus cuneatus
Fasciculus gracilis

Figure 4–10. Dorsal view of the brainstem and thalamus showing ascending somesthetic pathways. The spinothalamic tract is shown only on the left. The dorsal column system (including medial lemniscus) and the trigeminothalamic system are shown only for the pathways originating on the right side. VPL = ventral posterior lateral nucleus of thalamus; VPM = ventral posterior medial nucleus of thalamus.

In this way, sensory information from all portions of the body is brought to the ventral posterior regions of the thalamus: that from the face and oral cavity to the medial region (VPM); that from other portions to the lateral region (VPL).

E. Nontegmental Parts of the Brainstem

The tegmentum is the continuous central core of the brainstem; the nontegmental structures are discontinuous and separately appended to its dorsal and ventral surfaces. They are the **tectum, cerebral peduncles, ventral pons (pons proper)**, and **pyramids**.

1. Tectum

The roof of the midbrain is the **tectum**. It includes the **periaqueductal gray**, which is the gray matter surrounding the cerebral aqueduct (Figure 4–11). The tectum also contains a pair of **superior colliculi** and a pair of **inferior colliculi**, collectively called the **corpora quadrigemina** (Latin, four parts). The superior colliculi are concerned with vision, particularly visual reflexes, and receive much of their sensory input from the optic tracts. The inferior colliculi are concerned with audition and receive their input from large paired brainstem auditory tracts called the **lateral lemnisci**.

The axons from the inferior colliculi form the **brachium of the inferior colliculus**, which carries auditory information to the **medial geniculate body** (the auditory nucleus of the thalamus). There will be more on this in Chapter 7.

2. Cerebral Peduncles

Appended to—one could almost say hanging from—the ventrolateral aspects of the midbrain are the two **cerebral peduncles**, or **crus cerebri**. Their superficial portions are tracts containing a huge number of axons from the cerebrum. They carry information from the cerebrum to **nuclei**

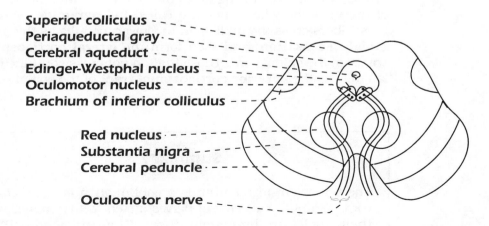

Superior colliculus
Periaqueductal gray
Cerebral aqueduct
Edinger-Westphal nucleus
Oculomotor nucleus
Brachium of inferior colliculus

Red nucleus
Substantia nigra
Cerebral peduncle

Oculomotor nerve

Figure 4–11. Cross-section through the superior colliculus of the midbrain.

in the ventral pons, to the inferior olivary nuclei, and to lower motor neurons of the brainstem and spinal cord.

The deeper portion of the crus cerebri, immediately adjacent to the midbrain tegmentum, is a very large nucleus called the **substantia nigra** ("black body," so called because its neurons contain a black pigment) (Figure 4–11). The substantia nigra is both structurally and functionally related to deep cerebral nuclei called the **basal ganglia**; it has a motor function that will be discussed along with motor speech mechanisms in Chapter 10.

3. Ventral Pons (Pons Proper)

A great many cerebral peduncle fibers synapse in the **pontine nuclei**, which are clusters of neurons deep within the **ventral pons**, or **pons proper**. The axons of pontine nuclei neurons cross the midline, form a large tract called the **middle cerebellar peduncle**, or **brachium pontis** (Latin, arm of the pons), and enter into the contralateral side of the cerebellum.

Some cerebral peduncle axons do not terminate on pontine nuclei. Many of these continue through the ventral pons on their way to the **inferior olivary nuclei**. Axons of inferior olivary neurons, you will recall, enter the opposite restiform body (inferior cerebellar peduncle) and carry information to the cerebellum.

4. Pyramids

Some axons of the cerebral peduncles pass through the pons proper without synapsing and emerge on the anterior surface of the medulla, where they are called the **pyramids**. Most of these fibers cross the midline in the lower medulla as the **pyramidal decussation**, and then form the **lateral corticospinal tracts** of the spinal cord. Those that do not cross continue ipsilaterally as the **anterior corticospinal tract** of the spinal cord.

Summary

The brainstem tegmentum is a continuation of the spinal cord. Ten of the 12 cranial nerves attach to the brainstem; their nuclei are brainstem nuclei. The oculomotor (III), trochlear (IV), abducens (VI), and hypoglossal (XII) are primarily GSE nerves. The vestibulocochlear (VIII) is a SSA nerve.

The trigeminal (V), facial (VII), glossopharyngeal (IX), and vagus (X) contain both SVE nerve axons and sensory fibers; they are thus mixed nerves. The spinal accessory (XI) contains only SVE axons. The nuclei of cranial nerves are discontinuous, unlike the continuous columns of nuclei in the spinal cord.

The reticular formation, inferior olivary nucleus, and red nucleus are also parts of the brainstem tegmentum. Somesthetic pathways pass through and from the brainstem to the ventral posterior lateral (VPL) and ventral posterior medial (VPM) nuclei of the thalamus.

Nontegmental portions of the brainstem are the tectum and cerebral peduncles of the midbrain, the ventral pons of the pons, and the pyramids of the medulla.

IV. CEREBELLUM

Although it is attached to the posterior surface of the pons, the **cerebellum** is entirely different from the brainstem, both structurally and functionally.

The cerebellum has two major functions.

- It coordinates muscle groups to orchestrate complex motor activity.
- It works with the vestibular system to coordinate the head's movements and static position with all other body activities.

All information entering and leaving the cerebellum passes through one or more of the three large cerebellar peduncles that connect the cerebellum and the brainstem (Figure 4–12).

- Proprioceptive information is carried to the cerebellum in the **dorsal** and **ventral spinocerebellar systems**. The axons of these spinocerebellar systems are part of the **inferior cerebellar peduncle (restiform body)** and part of the **superior cerebellar peduncle (brachium conjunctivum)**.
- Vestibular information is carried into the cerebellum, and from there back to the vestibular system, by a portion of the **inferior cerebellar peduncle (restiform body)**.

The anterior and posterior lobes are mainly involved in coordinating complex motor activity and the flocculonodular lobe in vestibular functions.

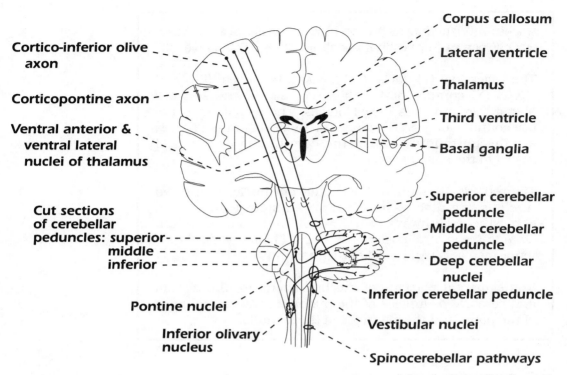

Figure 4–12. Schematic diagram of brain showing the basic neuronal pathways to and from the cerebellum.

- Cortical motor planning information is carried into the cerebellum by axons of the **pontine nuclei** that form the **middle cerebellar peduncle (brachium pontis)**; and by axons of the **inferior olivary nuclei** that course in the **inferior cerebellar peduncle (restiform body)** (Figure 4–12).
- Information from the cerebellum travels toward the cerebral cortex in the **superior cerebellar peduncle (brachium conjunctivum)**; it makes synapses in the thalamus, specifically in its **ventral anterior** and **ventral lateral nuclei** which, in turn, project axons to the **cerebral cortex**.

All information entering the cerebellum goes directly to the **cerebellar cortex**. This structure is composed of three elaborately organized layers of cells and covers the surfaces of all the **folia**; it is therefore extremely large. Proprioceptive, vestibular, and motor planning information is integrated in this cortex.

Cells in the cerebellar cortex send their axons to nuclei deep within the white matter of the cerebellum (Figure 4–12). Axons from these **deep nuclei** carry information from the cerebellum to other parts of the central nervous system—particularly to the vestibular nuclei and, by way of the thalamus, to the cerebral cortex.

Summary

The cerebellum coordinates muscle activity and functions with the vestibular system. Information to the cerebellum enters through the cerebellar peduncles and is processed in the cerebellar cortex; the cerebellar cortex projects the information to the deep cerebellar nuclei. The deep cerebellar nuclei project the processed information to the vestibular nuclei and to the cerebral cortex via the thalamus.

V. DIENCEPHALON

The **diencephalon** lies between the brainstem and the cerebrum. Its organization is different from that of all other parts of the brain. It has four portions:

- *The thalamus* is the largest portion.
- *The hypothalamus* is smaller; it lies ventral to the thalamus.
- *The epithalamus* is considerably smaller than the hypothalamus; it lies on the dorsomedial rim of the thalamus.
- *The subthalamus* is the smallest of all; it lies deep in the diencephalon between the thalamus and the hypothalamus.

A. Thalamus

Except for olfactory information and some input from the reticular formation, all information that goes to the cerebrum is first processed in the thalamus. It is composed of many structurally and functionally discrete nuclei (Figure 4–13). Some are especially important for the speech, hearing, and language scientist to know:

- *The medial geniculate body* is the auditory nucleus of the thalamus. On the brain's surface it appears as a bump at the end of the brachium of the inferior colliculus.
- *The lateral geniculate body* is the visual nucleus of the thalamus. It lies just lateral to the medial geniculate body and is at the end of the optic tract.

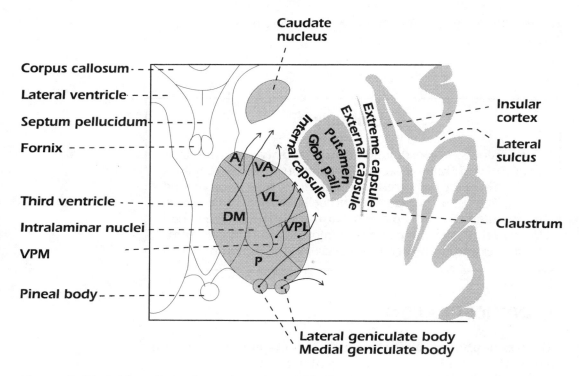

Figure 4–13. Schematic horizontal section through the thalamus and internal capsule. Arrows indicate axons of the thalamic nuclei entering the internal capsule. A = anterior nucleus of thalamus; DM = dorsomedial nucleus; P = pulvinar; VA = ventral anterior nucleus; VL = ventral lateral nucleus; VPL = ventral posterior lateral nucleus; VPM = ventral posterior medial nucleus; Glob. pall. = globus pallidus.

- *The ventral posterior lateral nucleus (VPL) and the ventral posterior medial nucleus (VPM)* are the somesthetic nuclei of the thalamus. They receive information from the trigeminal, dorsal column, and spinothalamic systems.
- *The anterior nucleus of the thalamus*, part of the brain's emotional circuitry, projects axons to the **cingulate gyrus**, which will be described in Section E at the end of this chapter.
- *The dorsomedial nucleus of the thalamus* is also related to emotional behavior. Its major projection is to the **prefrontal cortex** of the frontal lobes.
- *The ventral anterior and ventral lateral nuclei of the thalamus* (abbreviated VA and VL), receive information from the **basal ganglia**, and from the **cerebellum** via the **brachium conjunctivum**.
- Finally, there is a group of *intralaminar nuclei of the thalamus* that receive diffuse information from the **reticular formation** and from collaterals of other ascending axons.

As you see, each thalamic nucleus receives a specific type of information. The nuclei process the information and send it, via projection neuron axons, to the cerebral cortex. Each of these nuclei also receives information back from the cerebral cortex. The tract formed by these fibers, both coming and going, is a portion of the **internal capsule** (Figure 4–13).

The internal capsule, a huge tract, interconnects the thalamus and cerebral cortex. It also contains all of the axons that leave the cerebral cortex, bypass the thalamus, form the white matter of the cerebral peduncles, and go to brainstem and spinal cord levels.

B. Nonthalamic Parts of the Diencephalon

The nonthalamic portions of the diencephalon—**hypothalamus, epithalamus**, and **subthalamus**—are less important in speech, hearing, and language.

Recall that the hypothalamic sulcus in the **third ventricle** indicates the level where hypothalamus (ventrally) and thalamus (dorsally) juxtapose. The hypothalamus is primarily concerned with visceral functions such as hunger, thirst, and neural control of the endocrine system of hormones.

The epithalamus, composed of the **stria medullaris, habenula**, and **pineal gland**, lies on the dorsomedial rim of the thalamus. Its functions are unclear.

The subthalamus is structurally and functionally related to the **basal ganglia** of the cerebrum and will be discussed along with them in Chapter 10.

Summary

The diencephalon is composed of the thalamus, hypothalamus, epithalamus, and subthalamus. All information (except olfactory) reaching the cerebral cortex is first processed by thalamic nuclei.

The most important thalamic nuclei are the medial geniculate body (auditory), lateral geniculate body

(continued)

(visual), ventral posterior lateral and ventral posterior medial nuclei (somesthetic), anterior and dorsomedial nuclei (emotional), ventral anterior and ventral lateral nuclei (basal ganglia and cerebellum), and intralaminar nuclei (reticular formation). Thalamic nuclei project to and receive from the cerebral cortex via the internal capsule.

The other three parts of the diencephalon (hypothalamus, epithalamus, and subthalamus) are less important to speech, language, and hearing professionals.

VI. CEREBRUM

The cerebrum is composed of the two **cerebral hemispheres**. Each hemisphere has gray matter on its surface (**cerebral cortex**), white matter deep to the cortex, and large masses of gray matter still deeper (**basal ganglia**). In addition, each hemisphere contains a **lateral ventricle**.

A. Cerebral Cortex

As we have seen, the cerebrum is characterized by a superficial, convoluted cerebral cortex. In most parts of the cerebrum, this superficial gray matter is composed of six layers of cells and is called **neocortex**. In parts of the cerebral cortex that are evolutionarily older, there are only three layers of cells (**allocortex**); these are the cortices of the **cingulate gyrus**, the **septal region**, the **hippocampus**, and most of the **parahippocampal gyrus**. These three-layered portions of cerebral cortex comprise part of a functionally defined **"limbic lobe"** that is important in controlling emotional behavior. These portions are described in the last section of this chapter.

In each of the six layers of neocortex, there are distinct cell types and interconnections. The cells of the six layers are arranged into vertical columns, at right angles to the surface of the cortex and the plane of the layers themselves. This columnar organization is extremely important in the functioning of the cerebral cortex, as will be described in Chapter 8.

B. White Matter of the Cerebral Hemispheres

Lying deep to the cerebral cortex is a layer of white matter composed of myelinated axons whose sources and destinations vary widely. We can divide them into seven major groups, some of which can be subdivided into smaller groups.

- Axons that project up through the **internal capsule** to the cerebral cortex from cell bodies in the **thalamus**.
- **Short association fibers** with cell bodies in the cerebral cortex; the axons (fibers) dip into the white matter and then back up into the gray matter of an adjacent gyrus, forming a U-shape that gives them the secondary name of U-fibers. They communicate between nearby but separate regions of the cerebral cortex.
- **Long association fiber tracts** connecting distant portions of the cerebral cortex, usually in different lobes.
- The **corpus callosum**, whose fibers carry information between right and left cerebral cortices and thus keep them in constant communication with one another. This is the largest single tract in the brain.
- The **anterior commissure**—extremely small compared to the corpus callosum—which carries information between the anterior portions of the right and left temporal cortices. It also contains some crossing olfactory fibers.
- **Corticothalamic fibers**, which are the axons of cortical cells that project their information to thalamic nuclei.
- Axons of projection neurons of the cerebral cortex that bypass the thalamus and go directly to brainstem and spinal cord structures. These are:

So many groups of axons may be disconcerting now, but you will be meeting them all later on and they will make sense! Trust me.

Corticopontine fibers from the cerebral cortex, which pass through the **corona radiata, internal capsule**, and **cerebral peduncles** and terminate on **pontine nuclei** in the ventral pons;

Cortico-olivary fibers from the cerebral cortex, which pass down through the corona radiata, internal capsule, and cerebral peduncles and terminate in the **inferior olivary nuclei**;

Corticorubral fibers, which pass down through the corona radiata and internal capsule, dive into the tegmentum of the midbrain and terminate on the **red nucleus**;

Corticobulbar fibers from projection neurons whose axons leave the cortex and pass through the corona radiata, internal capsule, and cerebral peduncles. They terminate in **brainstem motor nuclei**: the GSE nuclei of cranial nerves III, IV, VI, and XII; and the SVE nuclei of V, VII, IX, X, and XI;

Projection cortical neurons of the **corticospinal system**, whose fibers form part of the corona radiata, internal capsule, and cerebral peduncles. They course through the ventral pons and form the pyramids. Most then decussate to form the lateral corticospinal tract on the opposite side; some continue on the same side and enter the spinal cord as the anterior corticospinal tract. Both crossed and uncrossed fibers terminate on **ventral horn motor neurons** of the spinal cord.

As these groups of axons pass to and from all parts of the cerebral cortex, they are called **corona radiata fibers**, a term that simply refers to their radiation throughout the crown of the brain (Figure 4–14). Then, between the thalamus and the basal ganglia, they become tightly packed to form the more compact structure called the **internal capsule**.

In this case, the term ganglion is unfortunate since a ganglion is a group of cell bodies in the PNS. However, in this case, basal ganglia are nuclei, not ganglia, and are part of the CNS.

C. Deep Gray Matter of the Cerebral Hemispheres

Deep within the cerebral hemispheres are large masses of gray matter (nuclei). The largest are the **basal ganglia**: the **caudate nucleus** and the **putamen**, which are functionally one nucleus split by the internal capsule; and the **globus pal-**

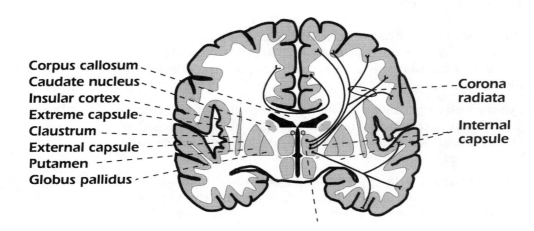

Corpus callosum
Caudate nucleus
Insular cortex
Extreme capsule
Claustrum
External capsule
Putamen
Globus pallidus

Corona radiata

Internal capsule

Figure 4–14. Coronal section through the cerebrum and diencephalon showing internal capsule and corona radiata and their relationship to other structures.

lidus, which lies on the medial aspect of the putamen (Figures 4–13 and 4–14).

The basal ganglia are part of a feedback circuit. They receive many axons from the cerebral cortex, process the information, and project it back to the cerebral cortex via the **ventral anterior (VA)** and **ventral lateral (VL) nuclei** of the thalamus.

Another deep cerebral nucleus is the **amygdala** (Greek for almond, its approximate shape), which lies deep to the cortex of the temporal lobe in the region of the **uncus**. The amygdala was formerly classified as a basal ganglion, but because it functions in affective (emotional) behavior, it is now regarded as part of the **limbic lobe** (see Section E below).

Finally, there is an area of poorly understood gray matter called the **claustrum** (Latin, closet), which lies just deep to the white matter below the **insular cortex** (Figures 4–13 and 4–14).

The **lateral ventricles**, filled with cerebrospinal fluid, also lie within the cerebral hemispheres: one in the right, one in the left. They are the largest of the brain's ventricles. The **body of each lateral ventricle** lies in the parietal lobe; the **anterior horn** extends into the frontal lobe; the **posterior horn** extends into the occipital lobe; and the **inferior horn** wraps from the body down into the temporal lobe. As already described, the lateral ventricles communicate with the third ventricle by way of the **interventricular foramina (foramina of Monro)**.

Deep in the temporal lobe there is some cerebral cortex that bulges into the inferior horn of the lateral ventricle and never reaches the surface of the brain. This is the **hippocampus**, which plays an important role in emotional behavior and in memory processing. It too is part of the **limbic lobe**.

D. Organization of Cerebral White and Gray Matter

The **internal capsule**, as we have seen, is a large fiber tract that contains axons carrying information between noncortical structures and the cerebral cortex. Two smaller capsules also carry fibers between noncortical and cortical structures. They are the **external capsule**, which lies between the putamen and the claustrum, and the **extreme capsule**, which lies between the claustrum and the insular cortex (Figures 4–13 and 4–14).

To get a mental picture of how these structures are arranged, recall that the insula is seen by spreading open the **lateral (Sylvian) fissure**. Imagine that you could journey from the lateral fissure through the **insular cortex**; you would encounter these structures, in the following order (Figures 4–13 and 4–14):

- **extreme capsule**
- **claustrum**
- **external capsule**
- **putamen**
- **globus pallidus**
- **internal capsule**
- **thalamus**
- **third ventricle.**

E. Limbic Lobe

As stated earlier, the **limbic lobe** is defined functionally, not structurally. However, there are definitive anatomical structures—cortices, nuclei, and tracts—whose complex neuronal processing and interconnections form the basis for our emotions.

The principal structures of the limbic lobe are:

- All three-layered regions of the cerebral cortex (**allocortex**)—**septal region, cingulate gyrus, parahippocampal gyrus**, and **hippocampus**;
- the **amygdala** of the cerebrum;
- the **mammillary bodies** of the hypothalamus; and
- the **anterior** and **dorsomedial nuclei of the thalamus**.

Tracts interconnect these structures in a complex manner, which we will explore in greater detail in Chapter 10. For now, it is enough to know that the allocortical structures, mammillary bodies, and amygdala project their information to the **anterior** and **dorsomedial thalamic nuclei**, which project to **prefrontal cortex** via the **internal capsule** and **corona radiata**. It is in the prefrontal cortex that our emotions interact with our perceptions, thoughts, and memories.

The limbic lobe in its entirety consists of a complex grouping of cortices, nuclei, and tracts. Although different parts of the limbic lobe have discrete functions, they all contribute to our emotions—joy, sorrow, motivation, love, hate and all the rest that tell us how we feel about ourselves and the world around us. As such they play important, often decisive, roles in our behavior, including what we say and how we say it. We will explore their roles in speech and language in Chapter 10.

Summary

Each cerebral hemisphere is composed of cerebral cortex, deep white matter, basal ganglia, and a lateral ventricle. Most of the cerebral cortex has six layers of cells and is called neocortex; a few portions contain only three layers and are called allocortex.

The white matter deep to cerebral cortex contains several fiber types, which are classified by their connections. These are:

- thalamocortical fibers
- short association fibers
- long association fibers
- corpus callosum fibers
- anterior commissure fibers
- corticothalamic fibers
- corticopontine fibers
- cortico-olivary fibers
- corticorubral fibers
- corticobulbar fibers
- corticospinal fibers.

The basal ganglia (caudate nucleus, putamen, and globus pallidus) interact with the cerebral cortex via the thalamus and are concerned with motor functions. The lateral ventricles extend into each lobe of the cerebrum. The limbic lobe includes both cerebral and non-cerebral structures concerned with emotions.

CHAPTER 4 SUMMARY

Information in the central nervous system is processed in nuclei and tracts with local circuit neurons and projection neurons; the information is carried to other parts of the CNS by tracts composed of the axons of projection neurons. Spinal nerves connect to the spinal cord via dorsal roots (sensory) and ventral roots (motor). In the spinal cord, sensory information is processed in the gray matter of the dorsal horn, and motor information is processed in the gray matter of the lateral and ventral horns.

Sensory information travels to the brain in discrete tracts of the spinal cord funiculi (white matter). Motor information travels from the brain to the gray matter of the spinal cord in discrete motor tracts of the funiculi.

The brainstem tegmentum is a continuation of the spinal cord, has cranial nerves III through XII attached to it, and contains the central nuclei of those cranial nerves. The cranial nerve nuclei are discontinuous as opposed to the continuous columns of spinal cord gray matter. The brainstem tegmentum also contains the reticular formation, the inferior olivary nuclei, and the red nuclei. Somesthetic pathways pass through and from the brainstem tegmentum to the thalamus.

Nontegmental portions of the brainstem are the midbrain tectum and cerebral peduncles, the pontine ventral pons, and the medullary pyramids.

The cerebellum is attached to the dorsal surface of the brainstem by the cerebellar peduncles. Information to be processed travels to the cerebellar cortex through these cerebellar peduncles. The processed information is carried to the deep cerebellar nuclei and then to the vestibular nuclei and, via the thalamus, to the cerebral cortex.

All information, except olfactory information, is processed in the thalamus of the diencephalon before it reaches the cerebral cortex via the internal capsule and corona radiata. The thalamus is composed of several discrete nuclei, each of which processes a different kind of information.

Nonthalamic portions of the diencephalon are:

- the hypothalamus for visceral functioning;
- the epithalamus, which contains the pineal body;
- the subthalamus, which functions with the basal ganglia.

Each cerebral hemisphere contains a superficial cerebral cortex with white matter deep to it, even deeper nuclei (the basal ganglia), and a lateral ventricle. Information reaches the cerebral cortex via the internal capsule and corona radiata. After it has been processed, the information can be:

- passed to other areas of cerebral cortex for further processing by short association pathways, long association pathways, and/or commissural pathways;
- sent back to the thalamus via corona radiata and internal capsule;
- sent to the basal ganglia via corona radiata and internal capsule;
- sent to the cerebellum via the corona radiata, internal capsule, and pontine nuclei; or
- sent to lower motor nuclei of the brainstem and spinal cord via corona radiata, internal capsule, and cerebral peduncles.

The basal ganglia are the putamen, the caudate nucleus, and the globus pallidus. They are involved in all voluntary, and many involuntary, motor acts. The limbic lobe controls and processes emotional behavior. Its structures include allocortical areas of the cerebral cortex and several noncortical structures of the diencephalon and cerebrum.

ADDITIONAL READING

Kandel, E. R., Schwartz, J. H., & Jessell, T. M. (1991). *Principles of neural science* (3rd ed.). New York: Elsevier.

Noback, C. R., & Demarest, R. J. (1962). *The human nervous system: Basic principles of neurobiology* (3rd ed.). Guatemala: McGraw-Hill.

Nolte, J. (1988). *The human brain: An introduction to its functional anatomy* (2nd ed.). St. Louis: C. V. Mosby.

Wilson-Pauwels, L., Akesson, E. J., & Stewart, P. A. (1988). *Cranial nerves: Anatomy and clinical comments.* Toronto: B. C. Decker.

STUDY GUIDE

Answer each question with a brief paragraph

1. Describe the organization of a spinal nerve.
2. Describe the gray matter and white matter of the spinal cord.
3. Which cranial nerves attach to the brainstem?
4. Which cranial nerves contain SVE fibers?
5. Describe the central nuclei of the vagus nerve including the functional role of each.
6. Describe the GSA nuclei of the brainstem.
7. What is the reticular formation?
8. Describe the central somesthetic pathways of the brainstem.
9. Describe the functions of the cerebellum.
10. What are the major nuclei of the thalamus?
11. What structures of the cerebrum have allocortex?
12. Describe the internal capsule.
13. What is the limbic lobe?

Odd One Out

In each of the following questions, choose the item that does not "fit" with the other three; briefly explain what the other three have in common that the odd one lacks. There may be more than one correct answer.

1. ____ general somatic afferent

   ____ general visceral afferent

   ____ special somatic afferent

   ____ general somatic afferent

   WHY?

2. ____ fasciculus gracilis

   ____ rubrospinal tract

   ____ spinothalamic tract

   ____ dorsal spinocerebellar tract

   WHY?

3. ____ oculomotor nerve

   ____ trochlear nerve

   ____ trigeminal nerve

   ____ abducens nerve

   WHY?

4. ____ facial nerve

____ glossopharyngeal nerve

____ vestibulocochlear nerve

____ vagus nerve

WHY?

6. ____ chief nucleus of V

____ descending nucleus of V

____ mesencephalic nucleus of V

____ motor nucleus of V

WHY?

8. ____ globus pallidus

____ amygdala

____ putamen

____ caudate nucleus

WHY?

5. ____ nucleus ambiguus

____ facial nucleus

____ nucleus solitarius

____ masticator nucleus

WHY?

7. ____ brachium pontis

____ brachium conjunctivum

____ brachium of the inferior colliculus

____ restiform body

WHY?

9. ____ red nucleus

____ inferior olivary nucleus

____ superior colliculus

____ inferior colliculus

WHY?

SECTION II

Balance and Hearing

Now that the fundamentals of Neuroscience are known to you, it is time to start a detailed look at the neural organizations that support communication. We begin with the mechanisms that receive and analyze sound—the most important sensory input (although vision is also important). And, oddly, we must also examine the sense of balance, not because it has anything to do with communication but because its peripheral and central structures are intimately connected and, therefore, must be understood and dealt with by audiologists.

In this three chapter section you will learn about:

- Peripheral and central vestibular mechanisms (Chapter 5);
- Peripheral hearing mechanisms (Chapter 6);
- Central hearing mechanisms (Chapter 7).

5

VESTIBULAR SYSTEM

Did you grow up thinking that there are only five senses: sight, hearing, taste, smell and touch? That common idea ignores several other senses whose receptors are diffuse and less obvious, such as pain, and one that has a prominent receptor organ, the vestibular sense.

Although we constantly use our vestibular sense, we are consciously aware of it only on those unhappy occasions when it malfunctions or is overstimulated. Then it commands attention: among other things it can cause vertigo, a hallucination of whirling movement often accompanied by nausea.

The hallucination may be that the environment is spinning, that you are spinning, or that both are happening simultaneously.

Under normal circumstances, however, the vestibular sense constantly sends information to the brain about the head's position and, when its position changes, about the speed and direction of change. This information is vital in maintaining visual fixation during head movements, maintaining balance through postural adjustments, and maintaining the proper relationship of head and body movements.

These three senses— vestibular, visual, and proprioceptive— are said to work synergistically: they interact with each other.

We now know that this adaptation involves anatomical and physiological changes in the central vestibular system.

Information about head position and movements is also provided by both vision and proprioception. Such redundancy indicates how important this information is from an evolutionary point of view. A person can usually get along with just two of these three senses. For instance, after a period of adaptation (up to 6 weeks), a person who has lost the vestibular sense can manage quite well as long as both vision and proprioception are functioning. However, in the dark, such a person becomes uncertain and may become disoriented and bump into things. Swimming, which decreases the amount of proprioception, is even more problematic; a person without a vestibular sense may have difficulty finding the water's surface and may even drown.

Many people have experienced adaptation in the vestibular system. For example, young children often suffer from motion sickness as a result of rapid horizontal acceleration and deceleration while riding in a car. To everyone's delight, their vestibular systems usually adapt to these forces over time and they outgrow the tendency.

I. PERIPHERAL VESTIBULAR SYSTEM

The **vestibular apparatus** is one part of the **inner ear**. (The other part is the **cochlea**; it is part of the auditory system and will be described in the next chapter.) The inner ear, whose longest dimension approximates the diameter of a dime, is a complex structure of interconnected, curving channels—hence its name, the **labyrinth**. It lies almost completely within the petrous portion of the temporal bone, which is the hardest, densest bone of the body.

The bone immediately surrounding the labyrinth is particularly hard and forms the **bony labyrinth**. Within the bony labyrinth is a fluid called **perilymph**. Chemically, perilymph is almost identical to cerebrospinal fluid, with a high concentration of sodium ions and a low concentration of potassium ions. It is continuous with CSF through a small channel.

In some people this channel is large; surgery such as a stapedectomy usually results in large flows of perilymph and CSF—called a "gusher" in surgical terms.

A. Parts of the Membranous Labyrinth

Suspended in the perilymph is another complex, hollow, fluid-filled structure, the **membranous labyrinth**. Strands of connective tissue fibers connect it to the inner walls of the bony labyrinth. The membranous labyrinth contains **endolymph**, a unique extracellular fluid whose chemical composition is similar to that of intracellular fluid (i.e., with a high concentration of potassium ions and a low concentration of sodium ions).

There is a higher concentration of potassium ions in endolymph than in any other part of the body.

Thus the membranous labyrinth contains endolymph and floats in a sea of perilymph that is contained in the bony labyrinth.

The posterior superior part of the membranous labyrinth is the **vestibular portion**; the anterior inferior part is the **auditory portion**, called the **cochlear duct** (Figure 5–1).

The vestibular membranous labyrinth is comprised of several parts (Figure 5–1). Prominent among them are three **semicircular ducts** on each side. Each duct has a swelling, its **ampulla**, that contains a patch of sensory epithelium called a **crista ampullaris** (Figure 5–2). The three ducts are oriented at right angles to one another. They are the **horizontal**, or **lateral, semicircular duct**, which lies at about 30° from the horizontal plane; the **superior**, or **anterior, semicircular duct**; and the **inferior**, or **posterior, semicircular duct**.

The ducts are interconnected with one another and with other structures of the vestibular system. One portion of the superior duct coalesces with one portion of the inferior to form a

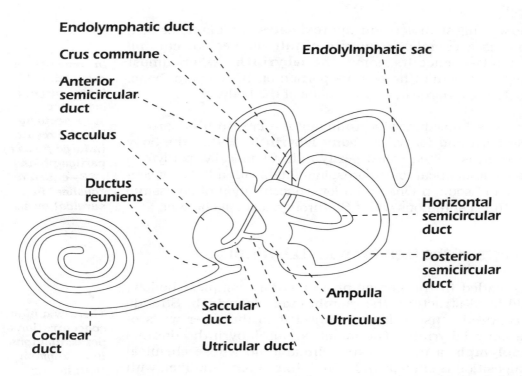

Figure 5–1. Schematic diagram of the lateral view of the left membranous labyrinth.

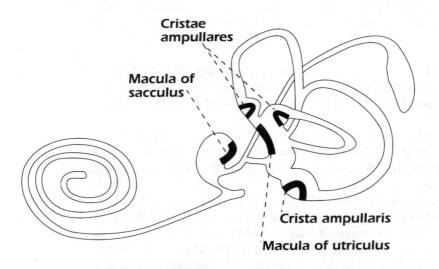

Figure 5–2. Same diagram as Figure 5–1, but also showing the locations of the vestibular sensory epithelia.

single duct called the **crus commune** (Figure 5–1). All three semicircular ducts are connected to a membranous epithelial bag called the **utriculus**; it contains a patch of sensory epithelium, the **macula of the utriculus** (Figure 5–2). Leading out of the utriculus is the **utricular duct**. It joins the saccular duct (described below) to form the **endolymphatic duct**.

The endolymphatic duct leaves the petrous portion of the temporal bone and expands into the **endolymphatic sac**, which lies within the meninges on the posterior surface of the petrous portion of the temporal bone. The other end of the saccular duct is continuous with another bag of endolymph called the **sacculus**, which is smaller than the utriculus. The sacculus also contains a patch of sensory epithelium, called the **macula of the sacculus** (Figure 5–2). The sacculus is connected to the cochlear duct by a narrow duct, the **ductus reuniens**—so named because it "reunites" the vestibular and auditory portions of the membranous labyrinth.

There is some evidence from experimental animals that the macula of the sacculus may also respond to some intense sounds.

B. Perilymphatic Areas Surrounding the Membranous Labyrinth

As explained above, the bony labyrinth contains perilymph that bathes all parts of the membranous labyrinth. Each semicircular duct is surrounded by perilymph and enclosed in a channel of the bony labyrinth; the duct and its perilymph-filled bony channel together form a **semicircular canal**. The sacculus, the utriculus, and their ducts are surrounded by a large well of bone-encased perilymph, the **vestibule**. Part of the vestibule's bony wall is the **oval window**, in which is embedded the **footplate of the stapes** (part of the auditory system) (Figure 5–3).

The perilymph in the vestibule is continuous with the perilymph in the **scala vestibuli** of the cochlea and, through it, with the perilymph in the **scala tympani** of the cochlea; this will be discussed in the next chapter.

C. Sensory Epithelium of the Vestibular Apparatus

The real work of this elaborate structure begins in the two types of sensory epithelia: the **cristae ampullares** (singular, **crista ampullaris**) in the semicircular ducts and the **maculae** (singular, **macula**) in the utriculus and the sacculus. Each of these epithelial tissues is composed of **hair cells** and **supporting cells** that hold them in place (Figure 5–4).

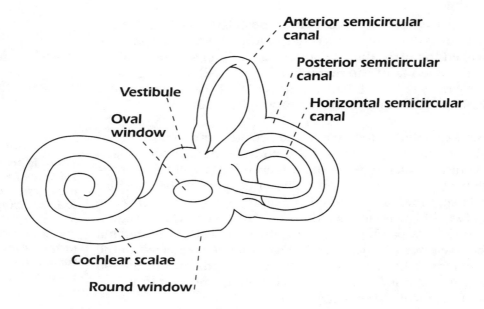

Figure 5–3. Schematic lateral view of the left inner ear perilymphatic spaces. The membranous semicircular ducts are within the semicircular canals. The utriculus, sacculus, utricular duct, saccular duct, and ductus reuniens are within the vestibule.

1. Hair Cells

Hair cells are the transducers of the auditory and vestibular sensory epithelia: they change mechanical stimuli into nerve impulses. They are the most sensitive mechanoreceptors of the body. In addition to the same organelles found in most cells, hair cells have several specializations for their particular role.

On all sides but one, the hair cells are in contact with perilymph—which is very similar, as we have noted, to the extracellular fluid that bathes all cells. On what we by convention refer to as the upper, or apical, end, the cytosol thickens to form a dense plate, called the **cuticular plate**. At the interface between endolymph and perilymph, the plasma membranes of the hair cells and supporting cells are so firmly held together that nothing can pass between the cells. These areas of cell adhesions are named **tight junctions** (Figure 5–4). Because of these tight junctions, perilymph and endolymph cannot mix. The chemical differences between these two separate environments play an important role in hair cell physiology.

Vestibular hair cells may be columnar or flask-shaped. The flask-shaped hair cells are also called **type I vestibular hair cells**: instead of small, bouton-type nerve endings on their

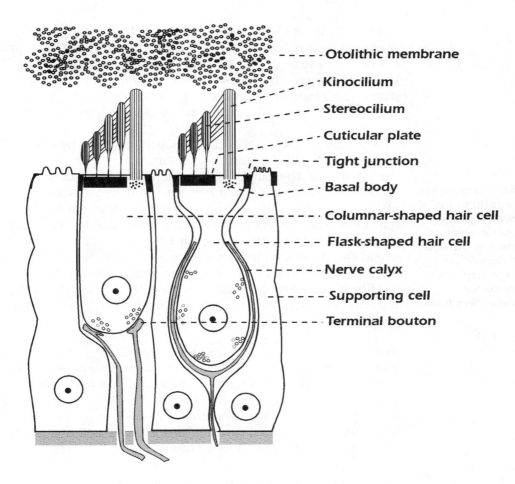

Figure 5–4. Drawing of two vestibular hair cells (a type I and a type II) showing their relations to three supporting cells, the otolithic membrane, and nerve endings.

base, there are extremely large synaptic endings that surround much of the cell. These unusual nerve endings are called **calyces** (singular, **calyx**). The columnar-shaped hair cells are called **type II vestibular hair cells**: they have normal bouton-type nerve terminals synapsing on their base.

From the apical ends of both types project two types of cilia: **stereocilia** and **kinocilia**.

There are usually over a hundred stereocilia on a single cell. Each is anchored in the cuticular plate by a narrow rootlet. Above the cuticular plate, each stereocilium is wider and contains many parallel molecules of **actin**—the same protein that in muscle cells combines with myosin to cause motion.

Note: hair cells do not have hairs like the hairs on your head. They do have stereocilia and kinocilia that protrude from the cells like hairs on your head—if your hair usually stands up on end.

There is only one kinocilium per hair cell. It is longer than the stereocilia and has no actin. Its root extends through an opening in the cuticular plate and ends in an organelle called the **basal body**, which lies in the cytosol deep to the cuticular plate. The kinocilium is eccentrically located, near the edge of the cuticular plate. This asymmetry polarizes the hair cell.

All the cilia on each hair cell are bound together by extracellular polysaccharides to form the ciliary tuft, which functions as a unit. When the ciliary tuft is bent in the direction of the kinocilium, potassium channels on the stereocilia are opened, allowing potassium ions to flow from the endolymph into the hair cells. The inflow of potassium ions excites the hair cells to release neurotransmitters at their base. The neurotransmitters excite the nerve endings that synapse on the base of the hair cells. These neurons then propagate action potentials along the **vestibular division of cranial nerve VIII** into the brain. Bending the ciliary tuft in the direction away from the kinocilium causes inhibition of the system.

The channels are actually pulled open by fine protein strands between the tips of stereocilia; these strands are called connecting links.

Note two important characteristics of this system. First, the ciliary tufts are extremely sensitive: even very weak forces will bend them and activate the system. Second, the system is directionally selective: bending in the direction toward the kinocilium excites the system and bending in the direction away from the kinocilium inhibits it. Intermediate positions give intermediate degrees of excitation.

2. Maculae of the Utriculus and Sacculus

The maculae of the utriculus and sacculus are structurally and functionally similar. Both are composed of supporting cells and hair cells. The stereocilia and kinocilium of each hair cell extend into the endolymph. The upper parts of both the stereocilia and the kinocilium are embedded in an **otolithic membrane**—a gelatinous structure that contains many small crystals of calcium carbonate (Figures 5–4 and 5–5). These crystals add weight to the otolithic membrane and enable it to respond to two types of stimuli:

These crystals are called otoconia or otoliths.

- **tilting of the head:** gravity pulls on the heavy membrane and bends the ciliary tufts, causing excitation or inhibition depending on the direction of the tilt.
- **rapid linear acceleration or deceleration of the head:** when the head moves, **inertia** delays the movement of the heavy otolithic membrane and that causes it to pull on the cilia. This is similar to what happens in an accelerating car:

Linear, in this case, means in a straight line.

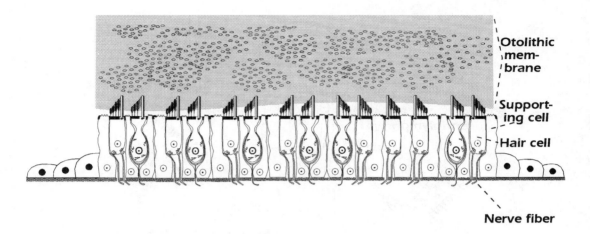

Figure 5–5. Diagram of a section through a portion of a macula of the utriculus or sacculus. Note that the kinocilia are oriented in opposite directions on the right and left sides.

when the car moves forward, you are pushed backward because your movement drags behind that of the car. If the brake is suddenly applied, the car stops faster than you do and your inertia thrusts you forward.

As stated, the hair cells are polarized by the placement of the kinocilium. Moreover, they are arranged in such a way that the kinocilia of half the hair cells of each macula "point" in one direction; those of the other half, in the opposite direction (Figure 5–5). In other words, half of the nerve fibers innervating a macula are excited by bending the head in one direction and half by bending the head in the opposite direction. Thus the maculae of the utriculus and sacculus provide the brain with constantly updated information about the head's resting position and rapid, linear movements.

3. Cristae Ampullares

The crista ampullaris of each semicircular duct is also composed of supporting cells and hair cells whose ciliary tufts extend into the endolymph. Each crista ampullaris rests on a mound of fibrous connective tissue (Figure 5–6). Its hair cells have long stereocilia and a kinocilium, all of which are embedded in a gelatinous membrane—in this case, a **cupula** —that totally blocks the semicircular duct. Unlike the otolithic membrane, the cupula does not contain otoliths and therefore has the same approximate weight and specific gravity as the fluid around it; therefore it does not respond to gravity. It does respond to *angular* acceleration and decelera-

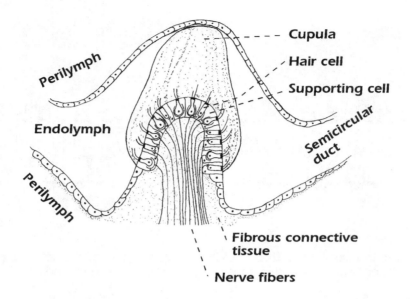

Figure 5–6. Diagram of a crista ampullaris. Note that the cupula occludes the semicircular duct.

tion, as described below, and gives the brain precise information about head movements.

The endolymph in the semicircular duct acts as a curved fluid column with inertia.

When head and body move together, it is a linear movement, detected by the maculae as described above. When the head moves relative to the rest of the body, the movement is angular, due to the way the head articulates with the vertebral column. The cristae ampullares are exquisitely sensitive to these angular movements, partly because of the curved column of endolymph in each semicircular duct. When the head is rotated in the plane of a semicircular duct, inertia causes the endolymph to lag slightly; this pushes on the cupula in the direction opposite to the rotation (Figure 5–7), and bends the ciliary tufts of the hair cells that are embedded in it. The bending of the ciliary tufts opens the potassium channels of the stereocilia, allowing potassium into the hair cells and activating them to release neurotransmitters; the neurotransmitters cause nerve impulses in the vestibular division of the VIIIth nerve. As in the maculae, the hair cells are direction-sensitive: they are excited when the cilia bend toward the kinocilium and inhibited when they bend away from the kinocilium.

Furthermore, the ducts on one side of the head are paired with those on the other side for complementary coding (Figure 5–8). To illustrate, the right superior and left posterior ducts are in the same plane and respond maximally to movements

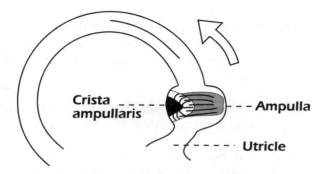

Crista ampullaris

Ampulla

Utricle

Figure 5–7. Schematic of a single semicircular duct. When rotated in the direction of the large open arrow, the inertia of the endolymph bends the cupula in the direction opposite to rotation (small, closed arrow).

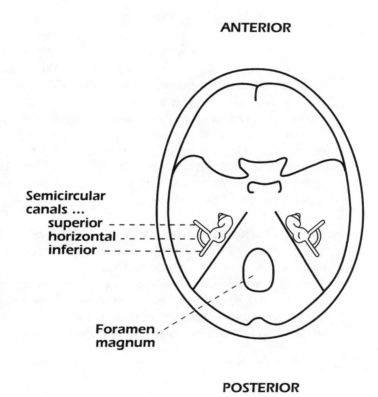

ANTERIOR

Semicircular
canals ...
  superior
  horizontal
  inferior

Foramen
magnum

POSTERIOR

Figure 5–8. Horizontal section through the skull looking down at the cranial cavity after removal of the brain. The locations and orientations of the right and left labyrinths within the petrous portions of the temporal bones are shown.

that are down to the right and up to the left; they respond to lesser degrees to movements that deviate from this plane, but such movements stimulate other canals to greater or lesser extents.

The combination of input from all six semicircular ducts gives very precise information about two important things:

A change in movement velocity is called acceleration if it is an increase, and deceleration if it is a decrease.

- the **direction of movement**, and
- the **change in movement velocity**—because it is when the head starts, stops, or changes velocity that the endolymph's inertia has its mechanical effect on the cupula.

Summary

The vestibular system senses the resting position of the head and any changes in head position. It functions synergistically with proprioception and vision. The membranous labyrinth is part of the inner ear and consists of several parts: (1) cochlear duct (the auditory portion), (2) sacculus, (3) utriculus, (4) three semicircular ducts, (5) endolymphatic sac, and (6) several interconnecting ducts (ductus reuniens, saccular duct, utricular duct, and endolymphatic duct). The membranous labyrinth is filled with endolymph and surrounded by perilymph.

The vestibular system has two types of sensory epithelium: the maculae of the sacculus and utriculus and the cristae ampullares of the semicircular ducts. Each sensory epithelium is composed of hair cells and supporting cells. The maculae respond to the static position of the head and to linear acceleration and deceleration. The cristae ampullares respond to angular acceleration and deceleration.

II. CENTRAL VESTIBULAR SYSTEM

The internal auditory meatus is the bony channel that carries the VIIIth cranial nerve.

The **vestibular ganglion (Scarpa's ganglion)** of the vestibulocochlear nerve is made up of the cell bodies of bipolar neurons that are the first order neurons of the vestibular system and lie in the **internal auditory meatus**. Their **peripheral processes** synapse with the hair cells of the maculae and the cristae ampullares (Figure 5–9). Their **central processes** form the vestibular division of the vestibulocochlear nerve. The cell bodies and peripheral and central processes are myelinated.

The vestibular division of the vestibulocochlear nerve enters the brainstem at the **cerebellopontine angle**. Most of its fibers synapse on second order neurons in the **vestibular nuclei**, which lie partially in the medulla and partially in the pontine tegmentum.

There are four nuclei on each side—the **medial, inferior, superior**, and **lateral vestibular nuclei** (Figure 5–10). The lateral vestibular nucleus, also called **Deiters' nucleus**, is character-

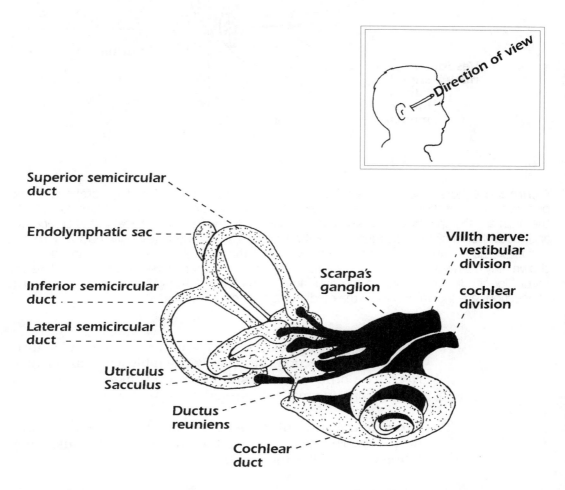

Figure 5–9. Innervation of the membranous labyrinth. (Simplified from a 1946 drawing by the famous biomedical illustrator, Max Brödel.)

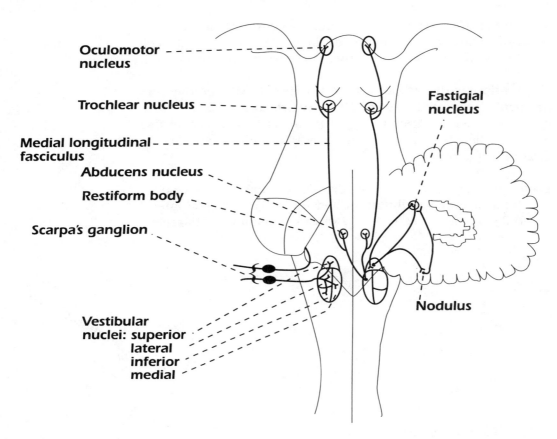

Oculomotor nucleus

Trochlear nucleus

Medial longitudinal fasciculus

Abducens nucleus

Restiform body

Scarpa's ganglion

Fastigial nucleus

Nodulus

Vestibular nuclei: superior
lateral
inferior
medial

Figure 5–10. Dorsal view of brainstem with part of the right half of the cerebellum. The positions of the vestibular nuclei are shown bilaterally. The connections of Scarpa's ganglion to the brain are shown only on the left. The connections of the vestibular nuclei to the cerebellum and motor nuclei of extrinsic muscles are shown only from the right vestibular nuclei. Note that all four vestibular nuclei project to and receive from the cerebellum, although connections are shown only from the superior vestibular nucleus. Similarly, all four vestibular nuclei project via the medial longitudinal fasciculus to the right and left nuclei of extrinsic ocular muscles, although connections are shown only from the medial vestibular nucleus.

ized by large, multipolar neurons with heavy Nissl substance; in histological section they closely resemble lower motor neurons. The other three vestibular nuclei, like most sensory nuclei, contain smaller neurons with less Nissl substance.

Axons of the vestibular nuclei neurons form several distinct pathways that can be considered six subsystems. They influence the following functions:

- **balance**
- **eye movements**
- **neck and head postural movements**

- **arm and leg postural movements**
- **nausea**
- **conscious awareness of vestibular sensation.**

The anatomical bases for each of these six functions are discussed in the next section.

A. Balance and the Cerebellum

Some primary and many second order vestibular central fibers project via the **restiform body** to two structures of the **cerebellar cortex** that make up the **flocculonodular lobe**—namely a lateral inferior structure called the **flocculus** and a midline structure called the nodulus—and also to the most medial of the **deep cerebellar nuclei**, the **fastigial nucleus**. These same structures send axons back to the vestibular nuclei (Figure 5–10). Because the cerebellum is the primary organ that synergizes all motor movements, this circuitry gives the vestibular system input to that process and promotes the coordinated movements that maintain the body's balance.

B. Eye Movements

If you move your head in any direction, your eyes automatically move in the opposite direction; thus you can simultaneously move your head and maintain visual fixation without thinking about it. The mechanism that does this is controlled largely by the vestibular system. Many neurons of vestibular nuclei project axons that synapse with the lower motor neurons of the extrinsic ocular muscles, which move the eyeball. These axons form the **medial longitudinal fasciculus**, often abbreviated **MLF**, a tract that lies just under the fourth ventricle and next to the midline; it extends from the vestibular nuclei to the motor nuclei of **cranial nerves VI, IV, and III** (abducens, trochlear, and oculomotor) (Figure 5–10).

When you consider that each eye is moved by six separate muscles, each of which must increase or decrease its tone by just the right amount for each reflexive movement, the neural complexity of this system is amazing.

This is a bilateral system: neurons of the right vestibular nuclei project axons to both right and left motor nuclei of cranial nerves VI, IV, and III; neurons from the left vestibular nuclei do the same. The cristae ampullares of the semicircular ducts detect not only all changes of the head's movement, but also their precise direction. This information, carried by the MLF to the motor nuclei of cranial nerves VI, IV, and III, controls the movements of the eyes relative to the movements of the head. This is called the **vestibulo-ocular reflex** (see the following box).

CALORIC TESTING OF VESTIBULAR SYSTEM

Some clinical testing of the vestibular system involves rotating the entire body, including the head, and measuring the eye movements. When the head and body are rotated to the left, the eyes move to the right; and when they have moved as far as possible, they rapidly move back to the left. This rapid return movement is called a **saccade**. The pattern—cyclic slow movements of the eyes in one direction followed by rapid movements in the opposite direction (the saccades)—is called nystagmus. If nystagmus is absent, or if its rate is either too fast or too slow, it indicates a vestibular disturbance. Such rotational tests are of limited value because they necessarily test *both* ears. However, peripheral vestibular disturbances are frequently unilateral, and a rotational test will not identify which ear is affected or if indeed both ears are affected.

A more frequently used test of the vestibular system is caloric testing. For this test a person's head is tilted back 60°, putting the horizontal semicircular duct in the vertical plane. Then the ear canal is douched with either warm or cold water. Because the horizontal semicircular canal lies close to the tympanic membrane, the douching cools or warms the endolymph of the horizontal semicircular duct, and sets up convection currents similar to what you would see when heating water in a pan. These convection currents stimulate the hair cells of the horizontal duct by pushing on the cupula and bending the ciliary tufts—much like what happens when the head is rotated in the horizontal plane.

The objectively observable result is horizontal nystagmus. With warm water douching, the rapid eye movements (saccades) are toward the ear being douched; conversely, with cold water douching, the saccades are away from the ear being douched. If there is no nystagmus in response to caloric testing, it means that ear's semicircular canal system is not functioning. Very rapid nystagmus to caloric stimulation means the semicircular canals of that ear are hyperactive. If one places recording electrodes on the skin around the eyes and records the electrical changes during eye movements on a chart recorder, one gets a permanent, objective record of the results of caloric testing. Such a procedure is called **electronystagmography**, usually abbreviated as **ENG**. In this manner each vestibular apparatus can be objectively and individually evaluated.

C. Head and Neck Movements

You use this reflex when you turn a corner while walking but keep your head and eyes pointed in the original direction.

An analogous mechanism, the **vestibulocollic reflex**, causes your head to rotate in one direction when your body rotates in the opposite direction (Figure 5–11). Axons of the medial vestibular nuclei form bilateral descending tracts—the **medial vestibulospinal tracts**—whose axons go to the lower motor neurons in the upper cervical region of the spinal cord. Thus the vestibulocollic reflex causes head movements without conscious awareness.

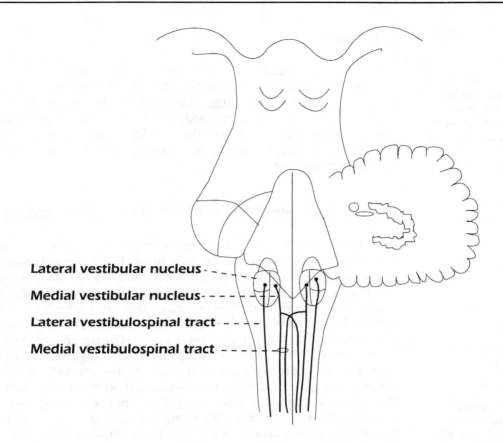

Figure 5–11. Dorsal view of brainstem with part of the right half of the cerebellum. The vestibulospinal pathways are shown.

D. Arm and Leg Postural Adjustments

The vestibular system provides the sensory input to the **vestibulospinal reflex**, which causes postural adjustments and thus keeps you from falling over when you lean far to one side. The axons of neurons in the lateral vestibular nucleus (Deiters' nucleus) form the **lateral vestibulospinal tract** (Figure 5–11). This tract terminates on ipsilateral spinal lower motor neurons whose axons pass to the extensor muscles of your arms and legs. Leaning over stimulates the maculae of the utriculus and sacculus, activating first order vestibular neurons that synapse on neurons of Deiters' nucleus. This information is carried via the lateral vestibulospinal tract to the appropriate lower motor neurons in the spinal cord, and activates them. They cause extension of the limbs on that side and keep you upright.

E. Nausea

Other brainstem nuclei, such as the nucleus solitarius, may also be involved.

Pathological changes, rapid spinning, or chronic rhythmic movements can overstimulate the vestibular system and result in nausea. Although the controlling neural mechanisms are not fully understood, we do know that collaterals of some axons of the vestibular nuclei go to an area of the brainstem called the **area postrema**, which is an **emetic (vomiting) center**.

F. Conscious Awareness of Vestibular Stimulation

As we have noted, we become consciously aware of the vestibular sense only when it is abnormally or excessively stimulated. It is not surprising, therefore, that its cerebral representation is quite small. Some axons from vestibular nuclei extend up through the brainstem and terminate in a **thalamic nucleus** that lies very close to the **ventral posterior complex**, which receives somesthetic information. Axons from this thalamic nucleus extend up through the **internal capsule** and **corona radiata** to a small cerebral cortical representation of the vestibular system that lies in the posterior inferior portion of the **postcentral gyrus**. A small portion of the **middle temporal gyrus** also responds to vestibular sensation, but there is no known direct thalamic projection to this area.

The ventral posterior complex is VPL plus VPM.

Summary

Vestibular hair cells are innervated by peripheral processes of bipolar neurons whose cell bodies form the vestibular ganglion (Scarpa's ganglion). Most of their central processes synapse with the vestibular nuclei of the brainstem. Some bypass the vestibular nuclei and join the axons of many vestibular nuclei neurons to terminate in the flocculonodular lobe of the cerebellum. The neurons of the flocculonodular lobe send their axons back to the vestibular nuclei.

The vestibular nuclei project axons that form the medial longitudinal fasciculus, which synapses with the motor nuclei that innervate the extrinsic ocular muscles. This is the anatomical basis for the vestibulo-ocular reflex. The vestibulocollic reflex is mediated by axons from the medial vestibular nuclei that form the medial vestibulospinal tract to lower motor nuclei in the upper cervical spinal cord. The vestibulospinal reflex is mediated by axons from the lateral vestibular nuclei that form the lateral vestibulospinal tracts to lower motor nuclei in the cervical and lumbosacral enlargements of the spinal cord. Nausea from overstimulation of the vestibular apparatus is mediated by axons of the vestibular nuclei that project to the area postrema. There is very limited cerebral representation of the vestibular system.

III. WHEN IT GOES WRONG

To better understand vestibular dysfunction, consider how alcohol in the bloodstream affects one's motor activities. For example, imagine that you and several companions have enjoyed the evening in a convivial bar on the top floor of a high-rise building. You are all at the point of feeling no pain. A keen observer might note that, when your friends do not deliberately fix their eyes on something, their eyes slowly drift in one direction and then rapidly return to the starting point. This is called **nystagmus**. It results from stimulation of the cristae ampullares by any of several causes—in this case, by the relative densities of alcohol and water.

If you are the nondrinking designated driver, you can entertain yourself by watching your friends' nystagmus.

Alcohol is lighter than water, the major component of blood and of extracellular fluids like endolymph. Therefore, as alcohol diffuses out of the capillaries, it sets up convection currents in the endolymph. These currents bend the ciliary tufts of the hair cells, which causes excitation, which initiates action potentials, which activate the vestibulo-ocular reflex, which causes nystagmus.

It is unlikely, however, that any of your party are aware of these events, or that they yet care.

Time comes to leave the bar. You walk to the express elevator—somewhat unsteadily, because this same stimulation of your semicircular ducts is sending strange and probably contradictory information to your central vestibular system. The elevator, a marvel of modern technology, plunges rapidly to the first floor. Added to the other challenges you have already presented to your vestibular system, this rapid descent might overstimulate your superior and inferior semicircular ducts, which could result in a profound feeling of nausea and possibly an embarrassing outcome.

Most people have never adapted to unusual vertical stimulation. Thus many adults get seasick—but seasoned sailors, who have had the opportunity to adapt, do not.

However, because you are a student of the nervous system, you know how to avoid this turn of events. You know that a lifetime of experience in automobiles has adapted your vestibular system to rapid horizontal acceleration and deceleration. Thinking quickly, you bend your head forward in a pious attitude, which aligns your horizontal canals with your present movement and minimizes the damage.

After reaching the street, the nondrinking designated driver gets you and your jolly companions to your respective homes. You clumsily disrobe, put on your pajamas, and head for the bed. Your companions, who do not have the benefit of your knowledge, probably leap into bed and turn out the light, only to sense the room spinning and their stomachs rebelling. You, however—student that you are—save yourself an agonized trip to the bathroom, because you understand that, of the triad of senses that provide information about one's position in space, two must be functional for their owner to be happy. Since you have temporarily messed up your vestibular system, you know you should give it minimal stimulation while you maximize input to your visual and proprioceptive systems, neither of which are affected by alcohol in the bloodstream. Therefore, leaving a light on, you *slowly* lie down, keep one foot firmly on the floor, and fixate on some object within your view. Soon you will go quietly to sleep.

Unfortunately, you will still have a hangover in the morning.

Another way to cope with the effect of alcohol on your vestibular system is to mix your drinks with heavy water (deuterium), using about two parts deuterium to one part alcohol. The heaviness of the deuterium compensates for the lightness of the alcohol and the drinks will not affect your vestibular apparatus. However, be aware that deuterium is expensive; each drink will set you back about $100 (plus the bartender's tip). And you're still going to suffer the morning after.

Perhaps there is an easier way.

Club soda, anyone?

Summary

When the vestibular system malfunctions, it causes spontaneous nystagmus, nausea, and vertigo. Mild forms of the same symptoms are caused by excessive intake of alcohol, because it has less density than water and therefore sets up convection currents in the endolymph. These currents cause chaotic stimulation of vestibular hair cells.

IV. VESTIBULAR SYSTEM AS A MOTOR SYSTEM

Consider this riddle: when is a sensory system a motor system?

The vestibular apparatus is a special sense organ and thus is the peripheral portion of a sensory system. However, stimulation of this organ causes motor responses that are reflexive and do not usually involve either thalamic or cerebral processing. This is in dramatic contrast to other sensory systems, in which the usual result of stimulation is cerebral awareness of sensation (i.e., consciousness) and possible reflex activity.

Thinking of it as part of a motor system that influences eye movements, neck movements, limb movements, and even visceral activity—rather than as a sensory system—adds an interesting perspective to the vestibular system.

CHAPTER 5 SUMMARY

The vestibular system, functioning in concert with proprioception and vision, provides the brain with information about head position and head movements. The peripheral vestibular system includes all of the membranous labyrinth except the cochlear duct and the perilymphatic spaces surrounding it. The maculae of the utriculus and sacculus respond to the static position of the head and to changes in linear velocity. The cristae ampullares of the semicircular ducts respond to changes of the head's angular velocity.

The neurons of the vestibular ganglion are bipolar. Their peripheral processes synapse with hair cells of the maculae and cristae ampullares. Their central processes form the vestibular portion of cranial nerve VIII and project to the vestibular nuclei of the brainstem. The vestibular nuclei neurons project axons to and receive axons from the flocculonodular lobe of the cerebellum.

The flocculonodular lobe and vestibular nuclei facilitate coordinated movements in response to vestibular stimulation, through several reflexes:

- **Vestibulo-ocular reflex**: maintains visual fixation while the head is moving. *Anatomical basis:* axons of vestibular nuclei that form the medial longitudinal fasciculus, which projects to the motor nuclei (VI, IV, and III); their axons innervate the extrinsic ocular muscles.
- **Vestibulocollic reflex**: causes compensatory head movements when the body rotates. *Anatomical basis:* axons of neurons in the medial vestibular nucleus that form the medial vestibulospinal tract to lower motor neurons of the upper spinal cord.
- **Vestibulospinal reflex**: causes postural adjustments when a body leans over. *Anatomical basis:* axons of the lateral vestibular nuclei that form the lateral vestibulospinal tract to lower motor neurons of the cervical and lumbosacral enlargements of the spinal cord.
- **Nausea**, caused by overstimulation of the vestibular apparatus. *Anatomical basis:* axons from vestibular nuclei to the area postrema.

Overstimulation of the vestibular apparatus results in spontaneous nystagmus, nausea, and vertigo. Normal functioning results in the active reflexive motor adjustments described, but little conscious awareness because there is little cerebral representation of the vestibular sense. Thus the vestibular system is more like part of a motor system than a sensory system.

ADDITIONAL READING

Cohen, B. (Ed.). (1981). Vestibular and oculomotor physiology: International meeting of the Bárány Society. New York: The New York Academy of Sciences.

Naunton, R. F. (Ed.). (1975). *The vestibular system*. New York: Academic Press.

Romand, R. (Ed.). (1992). *Development of auditory and vestibular systems 2*. Amsterdam: Elsevier.

STUDY GUIDE

Answer each question with a brief paragraph

1. What are the normal functions of the vestibular system?
2. Describe the structure of the membranous labyrinth.
3. Describe the functions of the horizontal semicircular canal.
4. What is the vestibule of the vestibular apparatus?
5. Describe the structure and function of the macula of the utriculus.
6. Describe the mechanisms involved in excitation of a hair cell.
7. Describe the vestibular ganglion and the structures its central and peripheral processes synapse with.
8. What is the role of the cerebellum in vestibular functioning?
9. Describe the vestibulo-ocular reflex.
10. What are the signs of vestibular dysfunction?
11. In what ways is the vestibular system part of a motor system?

Odd One Out

In each of the following questions, choose the item that does not "fit" with the other three; briefly explain what the other three have in common that the odd one lacks. There may be more than one correct answer.

1. ____ vision

   ____ audition

   ____ proprioception

   ____ vestibular sense

   WHY?

2. ____ cochlear duct

   ____ endolymphatic duct

   ____ saccular duct

   ____ superior semi-circular duct

   WHY?

3. ____ stereocilia

   ____ cuticular plate

   ____ dendrites

   ____ kinocilium

   WHY?

4. ___ vestibular ganglion

___ Deiters' nucleus

___ superior vestibular nucleus

___ medial vestibular nucleus

WHY?

5. ___ vestibular nuclei

___ medial longitudinal fasciculus

___ restiform body

___ flocculonodular lobe

WHY?

6. ___ vestibulocollic reflex

___ vestibulospinal reflex

___ medial vestibulospinal tract

___ upper cervical spinal cord

WHY?

7. ___ spontaneous nystagmus

___ nausea

___ vertigo

___ balance

WHY?

PERIPHERAL AUDITORY SYSTEM

Sound is defined as propagated vibratory energy. It can occur in gases, fluids, and solids. Hearing is the brain's perception of sound. Before the brain can deal with sound, it—like other sensory inputs—must be changed into nerve impulses. In this chapter you will learn how that occurs.

I. SOUND, SENSITIVITY, AND THE EAR

Sound can be described on the basis of three objective, physical, measurable parameters: **frequency**, **intensity**, and **duration**. In the process of hearing, each objective parameter is perceived as a subjective attribute. These perceived attributes are not exactly the same as the physical parameters but do relate to them.

- *frequency*—the number of vibrations per second, called Hertz (Hz), is perceived as **pitch**;
- *intensity*—the amplitude of the vibrations, measured in **decibels (dB)**, is perceived as **loudness**;
- *duration*—the temporal pattern of sounds, measured in seconds or tiny fractions of seconds, is perceived as the times when sounds stop, change, or start.

By adulthood, most people cannot hear above 15,000 Hz. This is not considered a hearing impairment.

A healthy young human can normally hear frequencies between 20 Hz and 20,000 Hz, although with aging the ability to hear higher frequencies decreases. The same healthy human can discriminate between frequencies that differ by as little as 0.2%.

We also hear over a wide intensity range, from sounds that are barely audible to sounds that are painfully loud; the latter are about a million times more intense than the former. Because this intensity range is so broad, we describe it in decibels, which are a logarithmic scale. In the frequency range we detect most easily—3000–4000 Hz (3–4 kiloHertz or kHz)—the amplitude of vibration of a barely audible sound is only slightly more than the random (Brownian) movements of air molecules. And we are able to discriminate between sounds whose intensity differences are as little as 1 decibel.

We also have very sensitive discrimination for duration, and can distinguish between two sounds whose durations differ by as little as 0.000006 of a second.

Summary

The physical characteristics of sound are frequency, intensity, and duration; their perceptual counterparts are pitch, loudness, and temporal patterns. Humans hear in only a limited frequency range (20–20,000 Hz, at best), but have a remarkable intensity range and excellent temporal discrimination.

II. PARTS OF THE EAR

We divide the ear into three parts (Figure 6–1): the **external ear**, the **middle ear**, and the **inner ear**.

The external ear is composed of the **pinna** and the **external auditory meatus**, an air-filled tube leading from the pinna to the **tympanic membrane (eardrum)**.

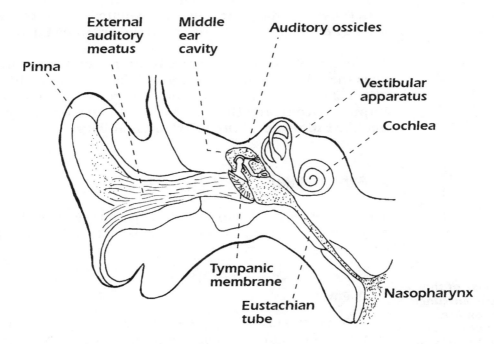

Figure 6–1. Coronal section through the ear showing the relationships of its major components.

The middle ear is an air-filled cavity, part of whose lateral wall is the tympanic membrane. It contains the **auditory ossicles**, three small bones that form a chain across the cavity and are named the **malleus**, **incus**, and **stapes** (Figure 6–1). They transmit sound from the tympanic membrane to the **cochlea**. The middle ear also contains two muscles: the **tensor tympani**, attached to the malleus; and the **stapedius**, attached to the stapes.

The entrance to the nasopharynx from the Eustachian tube is at a swelling named the torus tubarius.

The middle ear air space is continuous with the air in the **nasopharynx** through the **auditory tube**, or **Eustachian tube**. This tube is normally closed at its entrance to the nasopharynx.

The inner ear contains both the vestibular apparatus and the cochlea; the cochlea is the hearing portion (Figure 6–1). The cochlea is shaped like a snail shell, from which it derives its name. In humans, it has about two and a half turns. Sound enters the cochlea at its base, near where the **footplate of the stapes** is held in the **vestibule** of the inner ear. Because the inner ear is filled with fluid, the vibrations that were carried by the ossicles through the air-filled space of the middle ear must become fluid vibrations in the inner ear. These vibrations are then transmitted to the cochlea's sensory epithelium, which is called the **organ of Corti**.

The organ of Corti lies on the **basilar membrane**, which coils the full two and a half turns of the cochlea. Within the organ of Corti, physical vibrations are transduced into nerve impulses that are then carried into the brain by the **cochlear division of the VIIIth cranial nerve**.

A. External Ear

The external ear is composed of the pinna—good for holding eyeglasses and earrings—and the external auditory meatus, or ear canal.

Because of this elastic cartilage, you can bend your pinna and it will return to its original position and conformation when you let go.

1. Pinna

The pinna, or **auricle** (Figure 6–2), is made up of an elastic cartilage of irregular contours overlaid by skin. The muscles that move the human pinna are slight compared to those in mammals such as horses, dogs, or elephants, for whom pinna movement is far more significant. The pinna has only a minimal effect on hearing thresholds in humans.

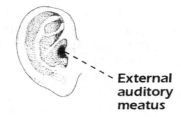

External
auditory
meatus

Figure 6–2. The human pinna. Its irregular contour causes high frequencies of sound to reflect differentially into the external auditory meatus, depending on the locus of the sound source.

However, if the pinna is bent out of its normal position—for instance, by being pulled forward—a person dramatically loses the ability to localize the source of a sound in the vertical plane (above or below one's head). To understand this, recall some physics of sound. High frequencies have short wavelengths; they reflect (i.e., bounce) off objects rather than refract around objects as low frequencies do. Unlike the pure tones of the testing lab, natural sounds are made up of a broad range of frequencies and always contain a considerable range of high frequencies. When high frequencies reach the pinna, they bounce off its irregular contours as if they were tiny ping pong balls. Some of the ping pong balls (sound energy) are bounced (reflected) into the external auditory meatus, where they can cause vibrations of the tympanic membrane (Figure 6–2). Just how many get there depends on the direction of the sound source. So if the pinna is distorted from its normal position and configuration, the pattern of high frequencies entering your external auditory meatus changes and your perception of the sound source is distorted. The pinna plays no other significant role in human hearing.

This can be easily demonstrated. Have a couple of friends pull their pinnas forward and close their eyes. Stand in front of them, jangle some keys, and ask them to point to the source of the sound.

2. External Auditory Meatus

The external auditory meatus is the tube, or canal, running from the base of the pinna to the tympanic membrane. It plays a significant role in hearing. The external auditory meatus is supported by cartilage in its outer portions (**cartilaginous external auditory meatus**) and by bone nearer the tympanic membrane (**bony external auditory meatus**). The skin that lines the tube is continuous with the skin of the pinna laterally and with the skin that forms the outer layer of the tympanic membrane medially. In the bony external auditory meatus, the skin adheres tightly to the bone. A hard object in the meatus will thus press the skin directly against the bone and stimulate pain fibers—a protective adaptation that helps keep foreign objects out of the ear.

The skin of the external auditory meatus contains hairs and two types of glands: one type, similar to sweat glands, produces a watery solution; the other produces a fatty solution. Ear wax, or **cerumen**, is a sticky substance formed by the mixture of the two solutions. Along with the hairs in the external auditory meatus, cerumen helps keep foreign objects away from the delicate tympanic membrane.

The external auditory meatus has a resonant frequency. Think of an empty soft-drink bottle: if you blow across its top, you produce a tone that is at its resonant frequency. If you add water (thus decreasing the effective volume), the resonant frequency, and thus the tone, will be higher. Although some people have a larger external auditory meatus than others, the resonant frequency of the human external auditory meatus is between 3000 and 4000 Hz .

Measurements demonstrate that a sound at the resonant frequency is 12 dB more intense at the tympanic membrane (i.e., after it has passed through the external auditory meatus) than it is at the base of the pinna.

This increase in intensity has clinical relevance. Excessive noise causes hearing loss. Although noise contains all frequencies, those that are most intense cause the worst damage. Because audiologists measure at octave intervals (e.g., 2, 4, and 8 kHz), the initial loss for noise-induced hearing loss is measured at 4 kHz and is called the **4k notch**.

In summary, the external ear facilitates vertical localization of sound; protects the delicate middle ear apparatus; and increases sound intensity by about 12 dB at the resonant frequency of the external auditory meatus.

B. Middle Ear

The middle ear is an acoustical transformer. It changes the air-borne vibrations that move the tympanic membrane into fluid vibrations in the cochlea. As always, to understand how this happens, we need to understand the anatomy.

1. Air Spaces

The middle ear contains two major and many tiny air spaces.

a. Middle Ear Proper: Tympanum The portion of the middle ear cavity nearest the tympanic membrane—the

middle ear proper—is called the **tympanum**. The tympanic membrane forms most of its lateral wall. The portion of the tympanum directly opposite the tympanic membrane is the **mesotympanum**; that extending below the level of the tympanic membrane is the **hypotympanum**; that above, the **epitympanum**, frequently called the **attic** (Figure 6–3).

      b. Antrum and Aditus ad Antrum A short tunnel, called the **aditus ad antrum**, connects the epitympanum with the **antrum**, a large air space within the mastoid portion of the temporal bone. Most of the rest of the mastoid portion of the temporal bone is composed of many narrow trabeculae (tiny spicules) of bone that contain among them numerous small air spaces called **air cells** (Figure 6–4).

There is great individual variation in the extent of air cells in the mastoid region. They often extend into the petrous portion of the temporal bone.

The tympanum, plus the aditus ad antrum and the antrum, plus the air cells throughout the mastoid portion of the temporal bone together create a large air space within the temporal bone, which is the **middle ear cavity**.

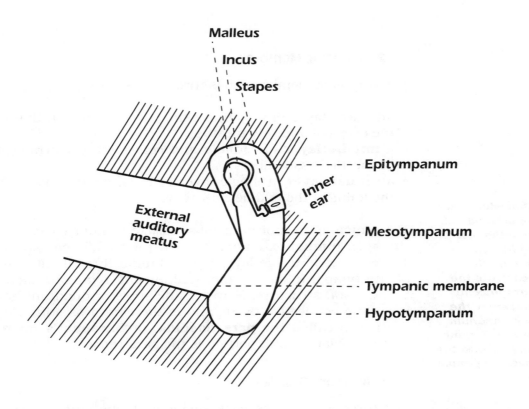

Figure 6–3. Diagrammatic coronal section through the middle ear showing the parts of the tympanum and the tympano-ossicular system. Hatching shows the adjacent parts of the temporal bone.

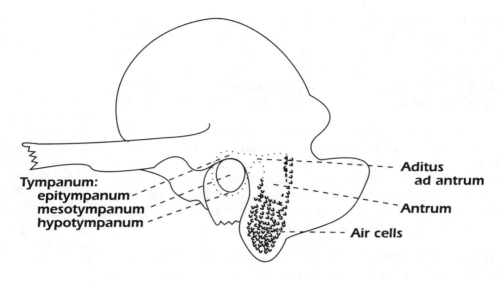

Figure 6–4. Lateral view of the temporal bone showing the positions of the parts of the middle ear cavity within the temporal bone.

2. Tympanic Membrane

The tympanic membrane has three layers:

- an **outer layer** of very thin skin, continuous with that of the external auditory meatus;
- a **middle layer** of radially and concentrically arranged connective tissue fibers;
- an **inner layer**, a single layer of cells, continuous with the lining of the middle ear cavity.

Cholesteatomas —pathological growths into the middle ear— frequently penetrate the pars flaccida and enter the epitympanum before growing further into the mesotympanum.

The tympanic membrane is shaped like a blunt cone, with the apex (**umbo**) extending toward the middle ear space. The connective tissue layer is substantial throughout most of the tympanic membrane, making the tympanic membrane a stiff structure. However, the superior quadrant has very little connective tissue and is therefore less stiff. This portion is called the **pars flaccida**, or **Shrapnel's membrane**; the larger, stiff portion is the **pars tensa**.

3. Auditory Ossicles

The three auditory ossicles—malleus, incus, and stapes— carry vibrations from the tympanic membrane to the inner ear (Figures 6–3 and 6–5).

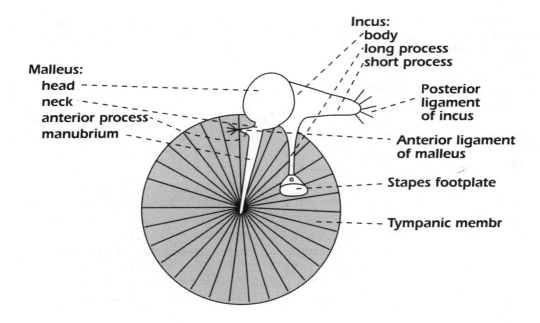

Figure 6–5. Medial view of the tympano-ossicular system.

The malleus is the largest. It has a long process, the **manubrium**, which extends from its narrow **neck** and is embedded along an entire superior radius of the tympanic membrane. The tip of the manubrium is at the umbo of the tympanic membrane; the manubrium is held within the tympanic membrane by fibers of the connective tissue layer. The head of the malleus lies in the epitympanum. Between the head and the manubrium is a short neck, at the base of which is the small **anterior process**; attached to this process is the **anterior ligament of the malleus**, which holds the ossicle in the middle ear cavity (Figure 6–5).

The head of the malleus articulates firmly with the **body of the incus**; there is no relative movement between them. The **short process of the incus** extends posteriorly from the body; the **long process of the incus**, which is parallel to the manubrium of the malleus, extends inferiorly from the body. At the end of the long process the bone makes a right angle turn medially and forms the articulatory process—named the **lenticular process of the incus**—which articulates with the head of the stapes.

The stapes is the smallest of the three ossicles. It has a **head**, and two **crura** (singular, **crus**) leading to the **footplate**.

An artery, the stapedial artery, courses through the obturator foramen during development. It is usually lost long before birth, but occasionally persists in adults.

Between the two crura is a hole, the **obturator foramen**. The footplate is held in the oval window of the inner ear by the **annular ligament**.

The chain of ossicles is suspended within the tympanum by two short, stout ligaments—the anterior ligament of the malleus, already mentioned, and the **posterior ligament of the incus**, which holds the short process of the incus to the posterior wall of the tympanum near the aditus ad antrum (Figures 6–5 and 6–6).

There are some other so-called "ligaments" (such as the superior ligament of the malleus); they are not true ligaments, being instead weak folds of the middle ear's mucosal lining that extend to the auditory ossicles. Despite their name, they are not stout enough to affect the vibrations of the ossicles. Their only clinical significance is that their geometry affects the growth directions of diseases such as **cholesteatomas**.

However, the anterior ligament of the malleus, the posterior ligament of the incus, and the annular ligament of the

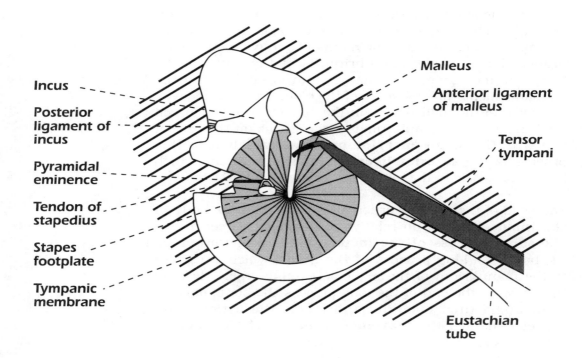

Figure 6–6. Medial view of the tympano-ossicular system showing the intra-aural muscles. Hatching shows the adjacent parts of the temporal bone.

stapes are true ligaments. An imaginary line drawn from the anterior ligament of the malleus to the posterior ligament of the incus defines the **axis of rotation of the ossicular chain**—and this holds one of the keys to the transformer properties of the middle ear. Because the manubrium of the malleus is embedded in the tympanic membrane, vibration of the tympanic membrane sets the whole ossicular chain into vibration. As the ossicles vibrate, they rotate around the axis of rotation. The manubrium of the malleus and the long process of the incus, which are parallel, form a lever apparatus whose long arm (the manubrium) is embedded in the tympanic membrane and whose short arm (the long process of the incus) articulates with the stapes. Among other things, these connections transform the vibrations at the tympanic membrane into piston-like vibrations where the stapes fits into the oval window. These piston-like vibrations in turn will cause perturbations in the cochlear fluids. The more closely the impedances of the tympanic membrane and the inner ear fluids are matched, the more efficiently the energy from the stapes vibrations will be transferred to the inner ear.

4. Impedance Matching Mechanism: Acoustical Transformer

Why is impedance matching so important? Consider what happens if you are swimming under water and your buddy in the rowboat shouts that a shark is approaching. The air-propagated acoustic energy of your buddy's agitated shout will reflect off the surface of the water rather than being transmitted to it. So you'd better have your eyes open because in this situation you are functionally deaf. In order to hear, you would need a mechanism at the air-water interface that would increase the sound pressure and/or decrease the volume velocity.

Such a mechanism is called an acoustical transformer—which is what the tympano-ossicular system is. It partially matches the impedance of air in the external auditory meatus with that of the fluids in the inner ear.

It does this by both increasing sound pressure and decreasing volume velocity at the oval window compared to the pressure and velocity in the external auditory meatus. Two mechanisms are responsible—an areal ratio mechanism and a lever mechanism.

Areal ratio: The surface area of the tympanic membrane is about 20 times larger than the surface area of the footplate

The same principle explains why your foot hurts more when it is stepped on by someone wearing spike heels than by someone wearing oxfords.

of the stapes. Therefore, although the *force* that moves the tympanic membrane and the force that is transmitted to the footplate of the stapes in the oval window are equal, the **acoustical *pressure*** is greatly increased at the oval window. This is because pressure equals force per unit area. Because of the differences in surface areas, the total force that moves the much larger tympanic membrane is concentrated onto the much smaller area of the footplate of the stapes and pressure is increased.

Lever system: The lever system, formed by the manubrium of the malleus and the long process of the incus, supplies additional amplification. The manubrium is about 1.3 times the length of the long process of the incus. A lever increases pressure at the shorter lever arm in proportion to the lengths of the two arms and, at the same time, decreases velocity to the same proportion.

In summary, the difference between the areas of the tympanic membrane and the footplate of the stapes increases pressure, and the difference between the lengths of the two lever arms both increases pressure and decreases velocity at the oval window.

These increases in pressure and the decrease in velocity at the oval window allow for weak air-borne vibrations to be efficiently transformed into fluid vibrations in the inner ear. However, the impedance matching is not perfect. A significant amount of the acoustical energy striking the tympanic membrane is reflected rather than transmitted to the tympano-ossicular system and thence to the inner ear. The following box quantitatively describes the impedance matching.

The efficiency of the tympano-ossicular system is also affected by its **mass** and **stiffness**. If the ossicles and tympanic membrane have large mass and little stiffness, they facilitate the transmission of low frequencies; if they have small mass and great stiffness, they facilitate high frequencies. The combination of mass and stiffness in the human tympano-ossicular system gives it a resonant frequency between 3 and 4 kHz—the same as that of the external auditory meatus. The tympano-ossicular system is most efficient in this resonant frequency range, and close to 75% of the acoustical energy is transmitted to the cochlea (see box, "Middle Ear Impedance Matching").

Because the resonant frequency of both the external auditory meatus and the tympano-ossicular system is in the 3–4

MIDDLE EAR IMPEDANCE MATCHING

Acoustical impedance increases as pressure increases and decreases as velocity increases. Another way to say this is that impedance is directly proportional to pressure and inversely proportional to velocity. In algebra this is expressed as

$$Z = \frac{p}{\mu}$$

where Z = acoustical impedance, p = acoustical pressure, and μ = volume velocity.

It is thus apparent that, because the tympano-ossicular system both increases pressure and decreases velocity, impedance is greater at the stapes footplate (oval window) than at the tympanic membrane. The extent of the impedance increase can be calculated if one measures the anatomical structures that contribute to the impedance increase. These are:

- area of the tympanic membrane (A_t)
- area of the footplate of the stapes (A_s)
- length of the manubrium lever arm (L_m)
- length of the incudal lever arm (L_i).

With these measurements, we can calculate the ratio of the impedance at the tympanic membrane (Z_t) to the impedance of the cochlea (Z_c) from the following equation:

$$\frac{Z_t}{Z_c} = \frac{A_s}{2/3 A_t} \left(\frac{l_i}{l_m} \right)^2.$$

Two-thirds of the tympanic membrane area (A_t) is used because about one-third of the sound energy reaching the tympanic membrane dissipates to the bone holding the tympanic membrane, leaving only two-thirds of the sound energy to move the ossicles. The lever ratio is squared because the lever system both increases pressure and decreases velocity, both of which increase impedance. When one enters the appropriate measurements of ossicles and tympanic membrane dimensions into the equation, one finds that the ratio of impedance at the tympanic membrane to that of the cochlea (Z_t/Z_c) is 0.0225. Physiological measurements of the cochlea demonstrate that Z_c (cochlear impedance) is 5600 acoustic ohms. With this, we can calculate the impedance at the tympanic membrane:

Since $\frac{Z_t}{Z_c} = 0.0225$

and $Z_c = 5600$

then

$Z_t = 0.0225 \times 5600 = 126$ acoustic ohms.

(continued)

The impedance of air, Z_a, in the external auditory meatus is 41.5 acoustic ohms, and transmission of acoustic energy from one medium to another is quantified as:

$$T = \frac{4\left(\dfrac{Z_t}{Z_a}\right)}{\left(1 + \dfrac{Z_t}{Z_a}\right)} = .74$$

What this means is that, at most, 74% of acoustical energy reaching the tympanic membrane is transmitted to the inner ear. It is actually less than that, since additional energy is lost due to factors such as frictional resistance in the tympano-ossicular system—for instance, at the ossicular ligaments.

Knowing the relationships between mass/stiffness and high/low frequencies can help you explain the anatomical bases for some conductive hearing losses.

kHz range, it is not surprising that human hearing is most sensitive in this range. At frequencies above and below this resonant frequency range, sound is transmitted less efficiently and hearing thresholds are higher. At frequencies below 3 kHz the tympano-ossicular system is too stiff for maximum transmission; at frequencies above 4 kHz, it is too massive.

5. Intra-aural Muscles

Recall that there are also two muscles in the middle ear—the intra-aural muscles.

The stapedius muscle is innervated by the facial nerve.

a. Stapedius   The stapedius muscle is the smallest discrete muscle in the human body. Its fleshy part lies within the bone of the posterior wall of the middle ear cavity; its tendon leaves through a small opening in a bony prominence called the pyramidal eminence (Figure 6–6). The tendon inserts onto the head of the stapes. When the stapedius contracts, it stiffens the ossicular chain, which reduces the transmission of low frequencies.

The stapedius is involved in two reflexes. In one, named the **stapedius reflex**, it contracts in response to a loud sound (over 80 dB hearing level). Because stiffening the ossicular chain reduces the transmission of low frequencies, and low frequencies have large amplitudes of movement, this reflex helps protect the inner ear from dangerously loud sounds that slowly intensify. Note, however, that it has no protective effect on sudden intense sounds—such as thunder or gunshots—that can permanently damage the inner ear before there is time for the stapedius reflex to act.

It is the reflexive contraction of the stapedius muscle in response to an intense sound that audiologists test with tympanometry (see box, "Testing the Reflexes").

The stapedius muscle also reflexively contracts just before vocalization and relaxes when vocalization is completed. Sound pressures in the pharynx caused by one's own voice often exceed 100 dB SPL (sound pressure level). This reflex protects our ears from being overstimulated when we speak so that we are ready to hear even faint sounds as soon as we stop speaking.

b. Tensor tympani

The second intra-aural muscle is the tensor tympani. It runs in a bony canal parallel to the wall of the Eustachian tube; its tendon extends out of the canal and inserts onto the upper part of the manubrium of the malleus. When it contracts, it both stiffens the tympanic membrane and pulls it toward the middle ear, thus slightly reducing the volume of the middle ear cavity. The tensor tympani functions in coordination with the tensor veli palatini muscle, which opens the Eustachian tube at its entrance to the nasopharynx.

These two muscles—the tensor tympani and the tensor veli palatini—work as a pair and are innervated by the same branch of the **trigeminal nerve**. Whenever we swallow or yawn, we simultaneously contract both, thus reducing the volume of the middle ear cavity and opening the Eustachian tube to the nasopharynx. This pushes any fluid that has accumulated in the middle ear cavity out into the nasopharynx. Under normal, healthy conditions, this phenomenon, called **middle ear clearance**, keeps the middle ear free of the fluid that slowly accumulates from the mucous membrane lining of the middle ear cavity. If the process fails to clear the middle ear and fluid accumulates, **otitis media** results. This may progress to an infection called **acute otitis media**, because warm fluids with little or no aeration are ideal breeding grounds for bacteria.

In infants, the middle ear clearance mechanism is not yet fully developed, which explains why infants so frequently have otitis media.

These actions of the tensor tympani and tensor veli palatini also equilibrate pressure between the nasopharynx and the middle ear. This "popping" of the ears relieves the feeling of pressure caused by altitude changes in a plane or a high speed elevator—although it was obviously not for these reasons that they evolved.

TESTING "THE REFLEXES"

An audiologist uses tympanometry to test "reflexes"—that is, the stapedius reflex. In this test, the external auditory meatus is sealed by a plug that creates a closed air space between it and the tympanic membrane. The plug, although making an air-tight seal, contains equipment to both produce controlled sounds and measure air pressure in the external auditory meatus. When a loud sound is played, the stapedius muscle reflexively contracts; this stiffens the ossicular chain and slightly moves the tympanic membrane. The movement of the tympanic membrane changes the air pressure in the sealed external auditory meatus. The tympanometer detects and records this pressure change and the audiologist knows that a reflexive contraction of the stapedius muscle has occurred.

This is an objective test involving the inner ear, middle ear, and part of the central auditory system. It can be done on infants and others who cannot verbally report what they hear.

C. Cochlear Anatomy

The cochlea transmits fluid vibrations from the stapes footplate in the oval window to the sensory epithelium of the organ of Corti. In the organ of Corti, vibrations are transduced into nerve impulses which, as you recall, are action potentials.

The cochlea is composed of three separate, fluid-filled columns—called scalae (singular, scala, Latin for stairway)—which coil two and a half turns around a bony, hollow core called the **modiolus** (Figure 6–7). The modiolus contains the **cochlear division of the VIIIth cranial nerve**; and the **bipolar cell bodies** of its neurons, which form the **spiral ganglion**. A ledge of bone—the **osseous spiral lamina**—spirals around the modiolus and is attached to it like a spiral ramp.

The three scalae are:

- the **scala vestibuli**, continuous with the vestibule, and filled with **perilymph**;
- the **scala media**, or cochlear duct, filled with **endolymph**;
- the **scala tympani**, also filled with perilymph.

At the apex of the cochlea is an opening called the **helicotrema**, through which the scala tympani and scala vestibuli are continuous (Figure 6–7). At its basal end the scala tympani terminates at the membranous **round window**, which faces the middle ear cavity. The round window membrane separates the perilymph from the air of the middle ear cavity.

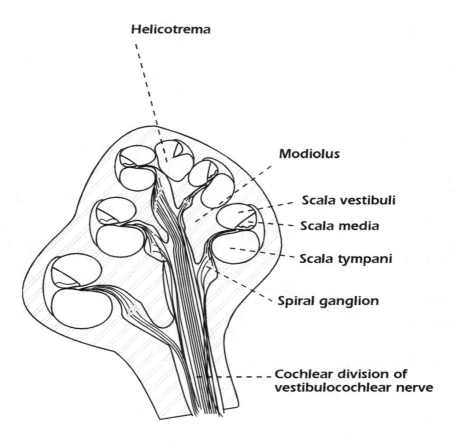

Figure 6–7. A section through the center of the cochlea through the length of the modiolus (called a midmodiolar section). Hatched areas are bone.

The perilymphatic scalae are completely separated from each other (except at the helicotrema) and from the scala media by membranes (Figure 6–8).

- **Reissner's membrane**, also called the **vestibular membrane**, separates the scala media from the scala vestibuli. It is very thin and is composed of flat cells.
- The **basilar membrane** separates the scala media from the scala tympani. It is a layer of radially oriented connective tissue fibers. On the scala media side lies the organ of Corti—the sensory epithelium of the cochlea.

The scala media itself, also called the **cochlear duct**, is completely lined by epithelial cells. They join one another in tight junctions, forming a barrier through which extracellular fluid cannot pass. Thus the endolymph and perilymph remain separate.

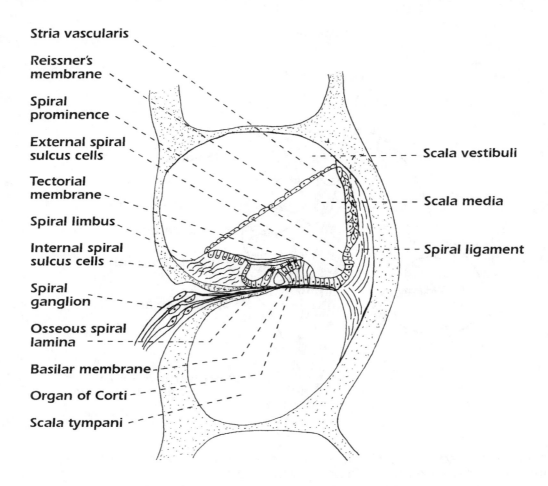

Stria vascularis

Reissner's membrane

Spiral prominence

External spiral sulcus cells

Tectorial membrane

Spiral limbus

Internal spiral sulcus cells

Spiral ganglion

Osseous spiral lamina

Basilar membrane

Organ of Corti

Scala tympani

Scala vestibuli

Scala media

Spiral ligament

Figure 6–8. A radial section through one turn of the cochlea. Stippled areas are bone.

Between the epithelium of the cochlear duct and the bone of the cochlea are three areas of fibrous connective tissue (Figure 6–8).

It is these radial connective tissue fibers that cause the stiffness of the basilar membrane. As you will soon learn, the stiffness varies with the length of the fibers and is important in frequency resolution.

- **Spiral limbus**: a ridge of fibrous connective tissue lying on the scala vestibuli surface of the osseous spiral lamina.
- **Spiral ligament**: an area of fibrous connective tissue against the outer bony wall of the cochlear turns. The lower part of the spiral ligament is opposite the scala tympani and the upper part is opposite the cochlear duct.
- **Basilar membrane**: radially arranged fibers that extend from the free edge of the osseous spiral lamina to the part of the spiral ligament that is at the level of the interface between scala tympani and the cochlear duct. It extends throughout the coiled length of the cochlear duct. On its

cochlear duct side is the organ of Corti; on its scala tympani side is perilymph.

1. Cell Types of Cochlear Duct

The epithelium of the cochlear duct is composed of diverse cell types (Figure 6–9).

Reissner's membrane extends from the spiral limbus at the modiolar side to the upper edge of the spiral ligament. Reissner's membrane cells are flat, and are called **squamous cells**.

Where Reissner's membrane reaches the spiral ligament, the epithelium changes dramatically. It becomes a structure

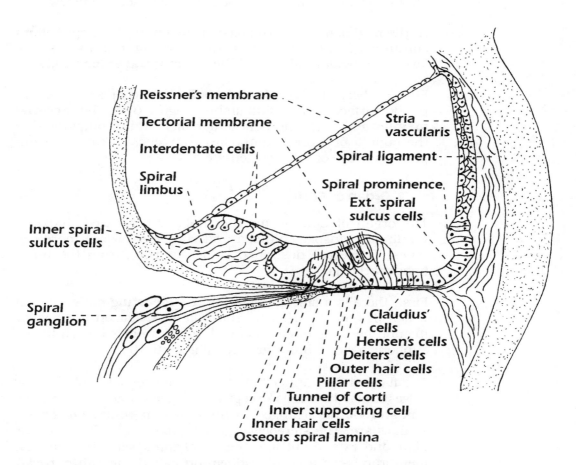

Figure 6–9. A radial section through the cochlear duct of one turn showing the cell types lining the cochlear duct. Stippled areas are bone.

The stria vascularis is the most metabolically active part of the cochlea. Therefore it requires a large blood supply.

called the **stria vascularis**, three cell layers thick and containing numerous blood capillaries, which give it the name. It lies against the spiral ligament externally and borders the endolymph of the scala media internally.

Just toward the basilar membrane from the stria vascularis, a modest outpocketing of cells bulges into the scala media: this is the **spiral prominence**.

A single layer of low cuboidal cells, called the **outer spiral sulcus cells**, extends from the spiral prominence to the organ of Corti (Figure 6–9).

The organ of Corti is the sensory epithelium of hearing. Most of it lies on the scala media surface of the basilar membrane; its innermost part lies on the surface of the osseous spiral lamina. Details of the organ of Corti are described below.

At the modiolar end of the basilar membrane, the epithelium continues along the edge of the spiral limbus as a single layer of cuboidal cells called the **inner spiral sulcus cells**.

Finally, there are **interdentate cells** on the upper, endolymphatic surface of the spiral limbus (Figure 6–9). The **tectorial membrane** (a gelatinous acellular membrane comparable to the cupula of a crista ampullaris) attaches to the endolymphatic surface of the interdentate cells.

2. Organ of Corti

The organ of Corti is more complexly organized than the vestibular sensory epithelia and contains several more cell types. These are described below, starting from the inner (modiolar) edge.

First, there is a single row of **inner supporting cells**, each of which lies on the osseous spiral lamina, not on the basilar membrane as is often assumed. Each inner supporting cell supports a single **inner hair cell** (Figure 6–10).

The flask-shaped inner hair cells are morphologically similar to vestibular hair cells except for the cilia. Each has numerous **stereocilia** arranged in three or four rows that form a shallow arc. The stereocilia all have rootlets in the cuticular plate and extend out into the endolymph below the tectorial membrane—an area of endolymph called the **subtectorial space** (Figure 6–10; see also Figure 6–13, page 192). During development, each inner hair cell also has a kinocilium, but

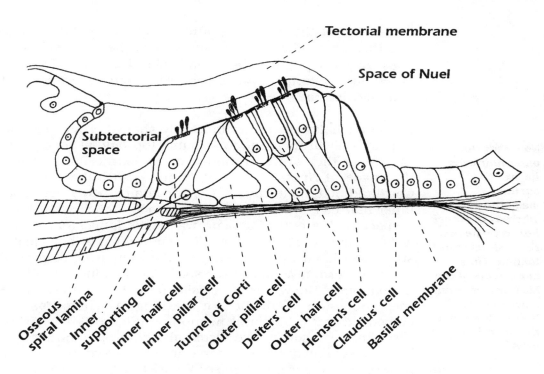

Figure 6–10. A radial section through the organ of Corti showing its cell types. Hatched areas are bone.

it is lost during maturation. Its original position is discernible as an open space in the cell's cuticular plate. The tallest stereocilia are in the row nearest where the kinocilium would be. About 18 sensory nerve terminals (boutons) synapse on the base of each inner hair cell.

Recall that vestibular hair cells each have a single kinocilium, even in adults.

Just beyond the inner supporting cells are two rows of **pillar cells—inner and outer**. Between them is a large extracellular space called the **tunnel of Corti**. The pillar cells have a strong cytoskeleton and give structural support to the organ of Corti. The inner pillar cell lies partly on the osseous spiral lamina and partly on the basilar membrane. The outer pillar cell lies entirely on the basilar membrane (Figure 6–10).

Beyond the outer pillar cells are three rows of **outer supporting cells**, or **Deiters' cells**. Each Deiters' cell has a cup-shaped depression that supports the base of an outer hair cell. From there, lying next to the outer hair cell, a narrow **phalangeal process** extends upward toward the endolymphatic surface of the outer hair cells and then expands. This expansion forms tight junctions with the apical plasma membrane of the adjoining outer hair cells (Figure 6–10). Together, the endolymphatic surfaces of the inner supporting cells, inner hair cells, pillar cells, Deiters' cells, and outer hair cells form an impenetrable surface called the **reticular lamina**.

Note that the outer hair cells lie over the basilar membrane, whereas the inner hair cells lie over the osseous spiral lamina. Thus movements of the basilar membrane move the outer hair cells but not the inner hair cells.

The outer hair cells are cylindrically shaped. They are held in place only at their endolymphatic "top" and at their base. Elsewhere they are surrounded by an extracellular space, the **space of Nuel**, which is continuous with the tunnel of Corti and, like the tunnel of Corti, contains perilymph. Like inner hair cells, the outer hair cells lack kinocilia but have a space in the cuticular plate where the kinocilium would lie (see Figure 6–12, page 190). Each outer hair cell has many stereocilia lined up in a few (usually four) irregular rows. The rows form a W-shape; the space for the kinocilium is at the bottom of the W The stereocilia in the row nearest where the kinocilium would be are the longest. Their tips are embedded in the tectorial membrane (Figure 6–10). A few very small sensory nerve terminals (boutons) and several large, vesiculated efferent nerve terminals synapse on the base of each outer hair cell (see Figure 6–12, page 190).

Between Deiters' cells and the outer spiral sulcus cells are three types of **border cells**:

- **Hensen's cells**, the tallest border cells, are adjacent to Deiters' cells;
- **Claudius' cells**, somewhat shorter than Hensen's cells, lie between them and the outer spiral sulcus cells;
- **Boettcher's cells** are found only in the basal turn; they are short cuboidal cells intercalated between Claudius' cells above and the basilar membrane below.

a. Tectorial Membrane   The **tectorial membrane** is an acellular, gelatinous membrane much like the cupula of the cristae ampullares. It is attached to the interdentate cells on the spiral limbus and extends out into the endolymph above the organ of Corti. The tips of the longest stereocilia of the outer hair cells are attached to its under surface. It has no contact with the inner hair cells (Figure 6–10).

D. Cochlear Physiology

Whereas the middle ear is an acoustical transformer that changes air-borne vibrations into fluid vibrations, the cochlea is an acoustical transducer that changes fluid vibrations into nerve impulses. This involves three consecutively occurring events:

- mechanical transmission of the sound from the stapes to the appropriate place along the cochlear duct;
- amplification of the vibrations at the most excited portion of the cochlear duct;
- transduction of the mechanical vibrations into nerve impulses;

and that's before it even gets to the brain where we understand and interpret what we've heard!

1. Mechanical Transmission of Sound

Sound is transmitted to the appropriate place along the cochlear duct because of the stiffness gradient of the basilar membrane. This structure is narrowest and stiffest at the base of the cochlea; it becomes increasingly wider and less stiff toward the apex (Figure 6–11). In fact, at its base the basilar membrane is 100 times stiffer than it is at its apex.

When sound enters the cochlea at the oval window, it sets the perilymph of the scala vestibuli in motion and starts a traveling wave that passes along the cochlear turns. When the traveling wave reaches the place along the cochlear duct where the basilar membrane's resonant frequency matches that of the sound that produced it, the sound energy passes from scala vestibuli through scala media and into scala tympani. This causes a vibration in a small area of the cochlear duct. Although these vibrations are very small, they are much larger than the extremely small vibrations over the area the traveling wave has traveled. Once the energy has passed through the cochlear duct at this place of matching resonances, the traveling wave stops; it passes no further apically. The energy, now in the scala tympani, is eventually dissipated at the round window membrane at the basal end of the scala tympani (Figure 6–11).

Recall that the oval window is in the vestibule of the vestibular portion of the inner ear, but it is continuous with the scala vestibuli of the cochlea.

Because of this stiffness gradient, the cochlea is tonotopically arranged: energy from 20,000 Hz sounds passes through the cochlear duct at its base; energy from 20 Hz sounds travels all the way to the apex before it can pass through the duct. Energy from intermediate frequencies passes through the duct in appropriate places in between. Energy from sounds below 20 Hz passes through the heli-

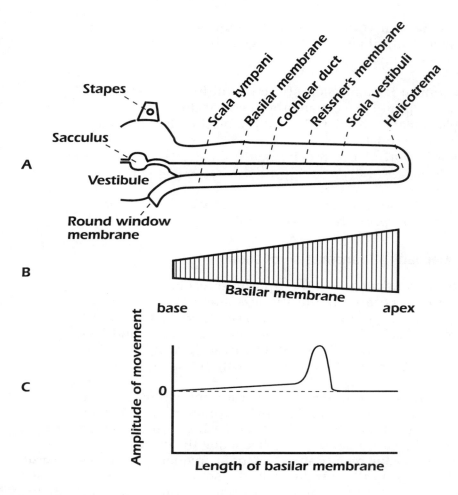

Figure 6–11. **A** is a diagram of the cochlea as if the spiral turns were straightened. **B** is a representation of a "straightened" basilar membrane showing its narrow base and wide apex. **C** is a graph showing the place of vibrations in response to a mid-frequency tone.

cotrema into the scala tympani without causing movement of the basilar membrane, which is too stiff to respond to such low frequencies.

This neat explanation contains a paradox that, starting in the late 1970s, inspired new investigations. Single hair cells in the cochlea and VIIIth nerve are sharply tuned: they respond with great sensitivity to a best frequency and poorly to frequencies above or below it. The mechanically driven traveling wave, which has low amplitude and a broad response, does not account for the sensitivity or frequency specificity of the auditory system. So what accounts for the exquisite sensitivity and specificity of the auditory system?

2. Active Amplification

Current experimental evidence indicates that the traveling wave induces an active metabolic mechanism that amplifies the energy at the best frequency. This **active process**, as it is called, is thought to result from activity of the outer hair cells.

Outer hair cells are shortest at the base of the cochlea and become progressively taller toward the apex. The stereocilia are also shortest at the base and tallest at the apex. The short outer hair cells at the cochlear base are tuned to high frequencies and the tall outer hair cells at the apex are tuned to low frequencies. In other words, the outer hair cells are tonotopically arranged just as is the basilar membrane. Moreover, the outer hair cells, surrounded by extracellular fluids, are able to move. When stimulated at their resonant frequency, they actually vibrate at that frequency, which greatly amplifies the movement of the basilar membrane at that specific point (Figure 6–12). This is believed to be the active process that sharply tunes the cochlea.

The mechanism of outer hair cell movements is not understood. We do know that it is different than the mechanism that causes muscle contractions.

When the basilar membrane moves up and down in response to the traveling wave and vibrating outer hair cells, it moves the portion of the organ of Corti that lies upon it, which pivots at the junction between the basilar membrane and the osseous spiral lamina. The tectorial membrane, driven by the stereocilia embedded in it as well as by fluid movements, also moves up and down. However, the tectorial membrane's pivot point is offset from that of the basilar membrane (Figure 6–10). Therefore the basilar membrane and the tectorial membrane do not maintain the same relationships during this movement as they do at rest. As a result, the joint but displaced movements of the two structures cause the stereocilia to bend, or shear, toward the outer wall of the cochlea and then back with each vibration. Naturally, the greatest shearing of the stereocilia occurs at the point where the stiffness of the basilar membrane and the tuning of outer hair cells are matched to the stimulating frequency.

This movement also produces eddies in the endolymph between the tectorial membrane and the organ of Corti (the subtectorial space). These eddies bend the stereocilia of the inner hair cells. The bending of the stereocilia of the inner hair cells is the final mechanical event in cochlear excitation, and the point where the transduction of mechanical vibrations into nerve impulses begins. (See box on "Otoacoustic Emissions" for an explanation of the effects of outer hair cell movements.)

There is some experimental evidence that the stereocilia of inner hair cells may contact the tectorial membrane during outer hair cell movements.

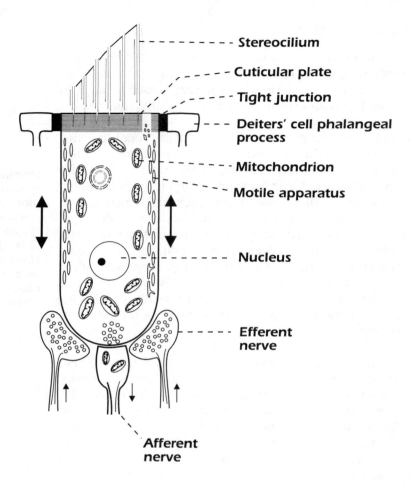

Figure 6–12. Diagram of details of a single outer hair cell and nerves terminating on it. When stimulated at its resonant frequency, it vibrates as indicated by the two-headed arrows.

3. Transduction

Although the physical properties of the cochlea determine how it mechanically transmits sound, its electrical-chemical properties determine the transduction process.

a. Resting Potentials Both extracellular and intracellular electrical potentials make the organ of Corti physiologically sensitive to mechanical stimulation.

The endolymph of the cochlear duct has a resting potential of approximately +80 mV at all times. This resting potential—called the **endocochlear potential**—is produced by the stria vascularis. It is most unusual in a biological system to have a positive extracellular electrical potential.

OTOACOUSTIC EMISSIONS

A sensitive microphone placed in the external auditory meatus near the tympanic membrane can detect sounds that are *produced* by the cochlea. Such sounds are called **otoacoustic emissions**. They are produced by movements of the outer hair cells—the same movements that actively amplify sound in the cochlea and are extremely sharply tuned.

Otoacoustic emissions are of three fundamental kinds:

- **spontaneous emissions**
- **evoked emissions**
- **distortion product emissions.**

When emissions have no apparent cause—that is, the hair cells appear to vibrate spontaneously—they are called spontaneous emissions. Frequent spontaneous emissions may be a sign of pathology. Evoked emissions occur in response to a brief auditory signal—essentially an echo of the signal. They are frequently called cochlear echoes. They have the same frequencies as the brief signal but at a much lower intensity. Distortion product emissions are a kind of evoked emission but contain at least one frequency not found in the brief signal. If two frequencies are simultaneously played to the ear, the distortion product emissions they evoke contain both frequencies plus some others, called distortion products, which are most prominent at the frequency $2f_1 - f_2$.

Otoacoustic emissions have become an important clinical tool. If outer hair cells are destroyed, not only is hearing severely depressed but otoacoustic emissions can no longer be evoked. It should also be noted that most sensory hearing losses involve the loss of outer hair cells. Because otoacoustic emissions can be objectively measured and require very little time, they are an excellent tool for screening populations for hearing losses—including infants. They can also be used to distinguish sensory from neural hearing losses.

Like all other cells, the outer and inner hair cells have **intracellular resting potentials** of about −60 mV.

Therefore, there is a difference in electrical potentials of approximately 140 mV between the endolymph and the inside of hair cells.

  b. Cochlear Microphonic The mechanical event of bending the stereocilia opens ion channels at the tips of the stereocilia, which causes potassium ions to flow from the endolymph through the stereocilia into the hair cells (Figure 6–13). That changes the endocochlear potential. Since the cause is an oscillatory, vibrating movement, the change in the potential is from positive to negative and back at the frequency of the stimulus. Thus an alternating bioelectric

Another bioelectric potential, the summating potential, can be recorded from the cochlea. Its functional significance remains unclear.

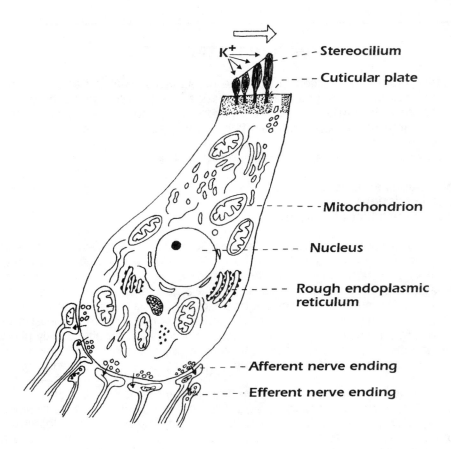

K+

---- Stereocilium

---- Cuticular plate

------ Mitochondrion

----- Nucleus

----- Rough endoplasmic
reticulum

----- Afferent nerve ending

----- Efferent nerve ending

Figure 6–13. Diagram of details of a single inner hair cell and nerves innervating it. When the stereocilia are bent in the direction of the open arrow, potassium ions (K+) flow through the stereocilia into the cell. This starts biochemical events that result in release of neurotransmitters at the base of the cell (small arrows).

current is created This is called the **cochlear microphonic**. Its frequency is the same as the sound causing it and its amplitude increases with sound intensity.

These biochemical events are currently being investigaged. We know they involve movements of calcium ions.

    c. Release of Neurotransmitter The flow of potassium ions into the hair cells causes biochemical events that result in the release of **neurotransmitter**—probably **glutamate**—into the synaptic clefts at the base of the hair cells (Figure 6–13). The neurotransmitter in turn depolarizes and excites the nerve endings of the VIIIth cranial nerve. When the depolarization is sufficient, it summates to action potentials traveling in the cochlear division of the VIIIth cranial nerve. This completes the transduction process.

Summary

The three major portions of the ear are the external ear, middle ear, and inner ear.

The external ear (pinna and external auditory meatus) allows for sound localization in the vertical plane, increases sound pressure by 12 dB in the 3–4 kHz range, and protects the middle ear from traumatic damage.

The middle ear consists of the middle ear cavity, the tympanic membrane, the auditory ossicles, and the intra-aural muscles. The tympanic membrane and auditory ossicles act as an acoustical transformer, changing airborne vibrations that move the tympanic membrane into fluid vibrations in the inner ear. This impedance matching mechanism increases the pressure and decreases the velocity of the footplate of the stapes relative to that of the tympanic membrane. The stapedius muscle stiffens the ossicular chain, which decreases transmission of low-frequency sounds. The tensor tympani and tensor veli palatini muscles function in clearing fluid from the middle ear and equilibrating pressure in the middle ear cavity.

The cochlea of the inner ear transduces fluid vibrations into nerve impulses. The cochlea has a central bony core, the modiolus, which contains the spiral ganglion and the cochlear division of the vestibulocochlear nerve. Three fluid columns (scala vestibuli, scala media, and scala tympani) spiral two and a half times around the modiolus. The basilar membrane is 100 times stiffer at the base than at the apex of the cochlea. Fluid vibrations in a traveling wave set the cochlear duct into vibration where its stiffness is matched to the vibrating frequency. This creates a tonotopic representation, with high frequencies basally and low frequencies apically.

The outer hair cells of the organ of Corti are also tonotopically arranged along the basilar membrane. They vibrate when stimulated, which amplifies the movements of the basilar membrane.

(continued)

> These vibrations of the basilar membrane and organ of Corti cause shearing movements between the outer hair cell stereocilia and the tectorial membrane. The movements of fluids in the subtectorial space cause bending of the stereocilia of inner hair cells. The bending of stereocilia opens the potassium channels of the stereocilia, and the influx of potassium ions results in the release of neurotransmitters from the hair cells which, in turn, excites the nerve endings synapsing with hair cells.

III. INNERVATION OF THE ORGAN OF CORTI

The organ of Corti is innervated by terminal endings of the cochlear division of the VIIIth cranial nerve. The innervation patterns of the inner and outer hair cells are quite different.

A. Afferent Innervation

All cochlear hair cells are innervated by peripheral processes of spiral ganglion cells. The central processes comprise the cochlear division of the VIIIth nerve, which terminates in the cochlear nuclear complex.

Although there are approximately three times as many outer hair cells as inner hair cells, 95% of the sensory fibers of the cochlea innervate only inner hair cells; in humans, about 18 spiral ganglion neurons synapse with each inner hair cell (Figure 6–14).

Outer and inner hair cells are similarly sharply tuned.

These are the **type I spiral ganglion cells**. Both their cell bodies and their peripheral and central processes are well-myelinated. Each is extremely specific in its sensitivity: it responds best to one frequency, and requires a much more intense stimulus for response to frequencies above and below that. A graph of frequencies against the intensity required to elicit a response from an individual nerve cell is a graphic representation of that neuron's tuning curve (Figure 6–15).

The other 5% of sensory neurons to the cochlea are the **type II spiral ganglion cells**. They are small, unmyelinated cells whose physiological properties are unknown because no one has been able to record from them. They go to outer hair cells, with each fiber making small afferent sensory synapses with many outer hair cells (Figure 6–14).

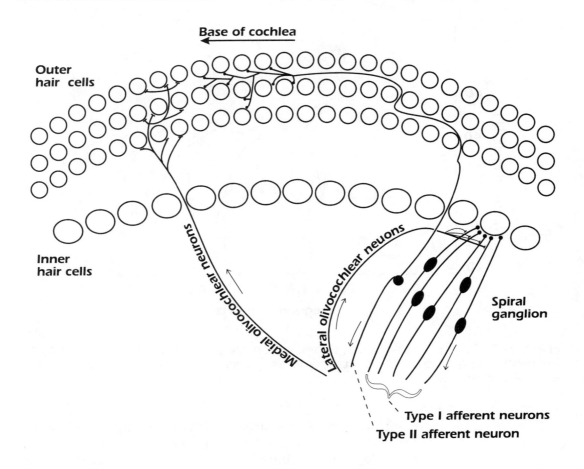

Figure 6–14. Diagram of the afferent and efferent innervation of the organ of Corti.

B. Efferent Innervation

The organ of Corti also receives efferent innervation from the **olivocochlear bundle (OCB)**. These are neurons with cell bodies in the **superior olivary complex** of the brainstem whose axons extend out to the cochlea. These neurons carry information from the brain to the ear instead of the reverse. In other words, the brain is controlling some activities in the cochlea.

You will learn much more about the superior olivary complex in the next chapter.

As is true for the sensory innervation, there are two types of olivocochlear bundle neurons: those that go to outer hair cells and those that terminate just under inner hair cells.

1. Medial OCB

Those that go to the outer hair cells form the **medial olivocochlear bundle**, so named because their cell bodies are in the

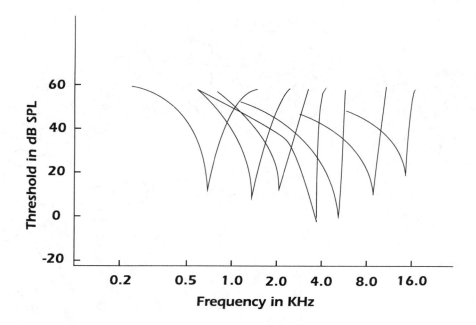

Figure 6–15. Tuning curves of seven spiral ganglion nerve fibers, each with a different best frequency. The graphs show the intensity levels in decibels necessary to excite activity in each nerve fiber as a function of frequency.

medial portion of the superior olivary complex. They are large neurons with well-myelinated axons. Most of the axons cross the midline to the opposite side of the brain and leave the brain with the vestibular division of the VIIIth cranial nerve; at the base of the cochlea they join the cochlear portion of the VIIIth nerve and travel within the spiral ganglion. Paralleling the afferent fibers, they then exit from the modiolus through the osseous spiral lamina and enter the organ of Corti, where they make large vesiculated synapses on outer hair cells (Figures 6–12 and 6–14).

2. Lateral OCB

The second group of olivocochlear fibers, whose cell bodies lie in the lateral part of the superior olivary complex, forms the **lateral olivocochlear bundle**. These are smaller neurons with unmyelinated axons that stay mostly on the same side and enter the vestibular portion of the VIIIth nerve. At the base of the cochlea they move to the cochlear portion of the nerve, travel within the spiral ganglion, and then pass out to the organ of Corti. They synapse just *under* the inner hair cells, on the peripheral processes of type I spiral ganglion neurons of the cochlea (Figures 6–13 and 6–14).

3. Functions of OCB

The functions of the neurons in the olivocochlear bundle are not fully understood. However, it is becoming evident that they are able to modulate the sensitivity of the cochlea, primarily in an inhibitory fashion. The medial olivocochlear bundle neurons appear to inhibit, or at least reduce, the movement of outer hair cells and thus reduce the sensitivity of the cochlea at that particular region. The lateral olivocochlear bundle neurons appear to influence the type I spiral ganglion peripheral fibers by making them more difficult to excite.

Although at first it may seem strange that the brain controls a part of our hearing, we have all experienced this many times. For instance, we often listen selectively to what we want to hear. At an orchestra concert, we can listen to just the violins, or just the flutes; at a cocktail party, we can listen to just the conversational partner of the moment.

Although the system did not evolve for the sake of concerts and cocktail parties, the ability to pick out an important sound in the presence of background noise can be a life-saving one. Think of hearing a predator in the forest or the cry of a baby in a windstorm. It is apparently the olivocochlear bundle that allows us to do that.

It is interesting that one of the biggest complaints people have about hearing aids is that they cannot select the signal—the important sound—from the noise, and have the most difficulty using the aids when they are in a noisy environment. This suggests that people with such hearing losses have lost or damaged their outer hair cells and thus the ability to suppress the things they do not want to hear.

Summary

About 95% of the spiral ganglion cells are large type I spiral ganglion cells. They innervate inner hair cells, with each inner hair cell receiving synapses from about 18 type I spiral ganglion neurons. The other 5% of spiral ganglion neurons are the small type II cells, each of which synapses with several outer hair cells. The organ of Corti also receives

(continued)

innervation from the brain via the olivocochlear bundle. Medial olivocochlear neurons are mostly crossed; they innervate outer hair cells with large, vesiculated boutons. Lateral olivocochlear neurons are mostly uncrossed and synapse with the peripheral processes of type I spiral ganglion neurons under the inner hair cells.

CHAPTER 6 SUMMARY

Humans can hear sounds in a limited frequency range (20–20,000 Hz at best), but they hear a wide range of intensities and can make very fine temporal discriminations.

The pinna of the external ear assists in the vertical localization of sounds. The external auditory meatus (also part of the external ear) protects the middle ear and resonates at 3–4 kHz, which increases the sound intensity at the tympanic membrane at these frequencies.

The middle ear acts primarily as an impedance matching transformer that changes the air-borne vibrations at the tympanic membrane to fluid vibrations in the inner ear. The tympanic membrane and auditory ossicles increase pressure and decrease velocity at the stapedial footplate relative to the tympanic membrane. This allows for partial impedance matching and the transformation of air vibrations to fluid vibrations.

Stapedius muscle contractions stiffen the ossicular chain, which protects the cochlea from intense low frequency sounds. The tensor tympani and tensor veli palatini muscles work together to clear the middle ear and to equalize air pressure between the middle ear cavity and the nasopharynx.

The cochlea transduces vibrations into nerve impulses. The cochlea has three columns of fluid (scala vestibuli, scala media, and scala tympani) that wrap around a central bony core (the modiolus)—in the human, for two and a half turns. Because the basilar membrane of the scala media is stiffest at the base of the cochlea and most flaccid at the apex, it gives the cochlea a tonotopic organization, with high frequencies received basally and low frequencies received apically. Sound energy passes through the cochlear duct (scala media) where the basilar membrane stiffness is impedance matched with the frequency of the stimulating sound. As the sound passes through the cochlear duct, it causes vibrations in the basilar membrane and organ of Corti. These vibrations result in bending of the stereociliary tufts of the hair cells. This bending opens potassium channels in the stereocilia; the resulting influx of potassium ions excites the hair cells to release neurotransmitters from their base. The released neurotransmitters in turn excite the sensory nerve endings that synapse on the base of the hair cells.

Type I spiral ganglion neurons comprise 95% of the sensory neurons innervating the cochlea. They innervate inner hair cells, with about 18 type I spiral ganglion cells synapsing on each inner hair cell. Type II spiral ganglion cells comprise the other 5% of spiral ganglion neurons. They innervate outer hair cells, with each type II spiral ganglion neuron synapsing on several outer hair cells.

The olivocochlear bundle forms an efferent pathway that carries neural information from the brain to the organ of Corti. Medial olivocochlear neurons, which are mostly crossed, innervate outer hair cells. Lateral olivocochlear neurons, which are mostly uncrossed, synapse with the peripheral fibers of type I spiral ganglion neurons just under the inner hair cells.

ADDITIONAL READING

Jahn, A. F., & Santo-Sacchi, J. (Eds.). (1988). *Physiology of the ear.* New York: Raven Press.

Pickles, J. O. (1988). *An introduction to the physiology of hearing* (2nd ed.). London: Academic Press.

Webster, D. B., Packer, D. J., & Webster, M. (1985). Functional anatomy of the external and middle ear. *Ear, Nose, and Throat Journal, 64,* 275–281.

Yost, W. A. (1994). *Fundamentals of hearing* (3rd ed.). San Diego, CA: Academic Press.

STUDY GUIDE

Answer each question with a brief paragraph

1. What are the physical parameters of sound?
2. Describe the structure of the external ear.
3. What auditory functions are carried out by the external ear?
4. Describe the functioning of the middle ear transformer.
5. Describe the mechanism of middle ear clearance.
6. Describe the modiolus and its contents.
7. Describe the epithelium of the cochlear duct.
8. Describe the tonotopic organization of the cochlea.
9. Compare and contrast the structure and function of outer and inner hair cells.
10. What are otoacoustic emissions?
11. Describe the afferent innervation of the organ of Corti.
12. Describe the efferent innervation of the organ of Corti.

Odd One Out

In each of the following questions, choose the item that does not "fit" with the other three; briefly explain what the other three have in common that the odd one lacks. There may be more than one correct answer.

1. ____ frequency

    ____ intensity

    ____ pitch

    ____ duration

    WHY?

2. ____ tympanic membrane

    ____ cartilaginous external auditory meatus

    ____ bony external auditory meatus

    ____ pinna

    WHY?

3. ____ mesotympanum

    ____ hypotympanum

    ____ epitympanum

    ____ antrum

    WHY?

4. ___ malleus

___ tensor tympani

___ incus

___ stapes

WHY?

5. ___ scala tympani

___ scala vestibuli

___ Scala media

___ vestibule

WHY?

6. ___ interdentate cells

___ inner hair cells

___ pillar cells

___ Deiters' cells

WHY?

7. ___ spiral limbus

___ spiral ligament

___ Reissner's membrane

___ basilar membrane

WHY?

8. ___ type I spiral ganglion cells

___ type II spiral ganglion cells

___ medial olivocochlear bundle cells

___ lateral oliv-cochlear bundle cells

WHY?

7

CENTRAL AUDITORY SYSTEM

The central auditory system consists of the **auditory brainstem**, which includes several auditory pathways, and the **auditory forebrain**.

The auditory brainstem is more than just a collection of nuclei and tracts that relay auditory signals from the ear to the thalamus and thence to the cerebral cortex. It is composed of processing centers, arranged both serially and in parallel, where auditory signals are analyzed and coded to transmit sophisticated information.

The cochlea transduces sound into action potentials coded for frequency, intensity, and temporal information. The cochlear division of the **vestibulocochlear nerve** carries these impulses into the brainstem, where they undergo further processing. Although this processing involves a large number of tracts and nuclei, the coding for frequency, intensity, and temporal information is maintained. Many of the structures involved in this processing are commonly referred to by abbreviations; they are summarized in the box on page 205.

I. COCHLEAR NUCLEAR COMPLEX

The **cochlear nuclear complex** spans the border between pons and medulla at the **cerebellopontine angle**. It is morphologically and physiologically divisible into two portions: the **dorsal cochlear nucleus (DCN)** and the **ventral cochlear nucleus (VCN)**. The latter is further divided into **anterior ventral cochlear nucleus (AVCN)** and **posterior ventral cochlear nucleus (PVCN)** (Figure 7–1). It is possible to further subdivide the cochlear nuclear complex (see the box on parcellation), but for our purposes it is not necessary to do so.

Note that each primary neuron synapses with several second order neurons, which facilitates central processing.

The central fibers of both type I and type II **spiral ganglion neurons** bifurcate in VCN. An **ascending branch** goes to AVCN; a **descending branch** goes first to PVCN and then to DCN. Individual ascending and descending branches may each synapse with several neurons of the cochlear nuclear complex.

Type I spiral ganglion fibers are coded for frequency by their sharp tuning curves: that is, they respond with great sensitivity to an extremely narrow band of frequencies and

ALPHABET SOUP

AVCN	Anterior ventral cochlear nucleus
CNIC	Central nucleus of the inferior colliculus
DCN	Dorsal cochlear nucleus
DNLL	Dorsal nucleus of the lateral lemniscus
LSO	Lateral superior olivary nucleus; lateral superior olive
MNTB	Medial nucleus of the trapezoid body
MSO	Medial superior olivary nucleus; medial superior olive
PVCN	Posterior ventral cochlear nucleus
SOC	Superior olivary complex
Stria of Held	Intermediate acoustic stria
Stria of Monakow	Dorsal acoustic stria
VCN	Ventral cochlear nucleus
VIIth cranial nerve	Facial nerve
VIIIth cranial nerve	Vestibulocochlear nerve
VNLL	Ventral nucleus of the lateral lemniscus

are much less sensitive to frequencies just above and below this best frequency.

Type I fibers are also coded for intensity: the more intense the stimulating sound, the more nerve impulses the fibers conduct per unit of time.

Type II fibers are a mystery. No one has been able to record physiological activity from them. In fact, it has been suggested that type II fibers, which have very small diameters, no myelin sheaths, and long trajectories, do not conduct nerve impulses.

The central fibers of both type I and type II spiral ganglion neurons are distributed throughout the three divisions of the cochlear nuclear complex in *cochleotopic*, and thus *tonotopic*, arrangements:

- Low frequency fibers, from the apex of the cochlea, bifurcate almost immediately upon entering the cochlear nuclei. An ascending branch goes to the ventrolateral portion of AVCN; a descending branch goes to the ventrolateral portions of both PVCN and DCN.

The tonotopic organization is repeated in most, if not all, auditory nuclei and cortices.

PARCELLATION OF THE COCHLEAR NUCLEAR COMPLEX

Anatomists realized in the late 19th century that cochlear nerve fibers enter the brain, bifurcate into ascending and descending branches, and synapse on second order cells.

Those second order cells were later defined as the cochlear nuclear complex. In the early 20th century, the complex was parcellated into three subdivisions, defined by the fibers synapsing in each.

- Ascending fibers synapse on cells of the anterior ventral cochlear nucleus (AVCN).
- Descending fibers synapse first on cells of the posterior ventral cochlear nucleus (PVCN).
- Descending fibers then synapse on a layered structure, the dorsal cochlear nucleus (DCN).

By the middle of the 20th century, it was also recognized that each of these subdivisions, or nuclei, contains different cell types.

Thanks to new microscopic techniques and devices, scientists have been able to look even more closely at both the architecture of the complex and its cell types.

Using a variety of organizational schemes, some investigators have split each nucleus into smaller and smaller cytoarchitectonic units, describing as many as 30 different areas within the complex. Many of these subdivisions are difficult to identify; as far as we know, many are not physiological entities. Moreover, the experts themselves do not agree on their definitions.

Other investigators, myself included, have looked at cells and described over 20 specific types within the complex. These definitions have been based on interpretations of cell size, cell body shape, and the extent and directions of dendritic branches.

The result is a literature in which variants of cell types are named as new cell types, the same cells are called by different names, and either the nuclei are split into small subdivisions or their subdivisions are lumped together into larger units—in short, a literature as complex as the structures themselves and a challenge for all but the most dedicated anatomists to read.

When in Doubt, Consult the Classics

To help us find a path through this morass of contradictory detail, this book uses the early 20th century scheme. We will divide the cochlear nuclear complex into the standard three major nuclei. In each nucleus we will be concerned only with the prominent, distinctive cell types, whose physiology is also at least partially understood. Thus, of the more than 20 cell types that have been described, we will deal with only five: in AVCN, the globular and spherical bushy cells; in PVCN, the octopus cells; in DCN, the stellate cells; and throughout both AVCN and PVCN, the multipolar cells.

This simplified scheme will help improve understanding without distorting the basic organization. We will use similar simplified schemes in discussing other nuclei and tracts.

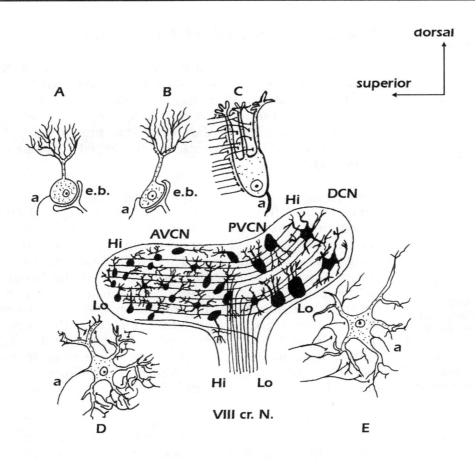

dorsal

superior

Figure 7–1. Diagrammatic parasagittal section through the cochlear nuclear complex and cochlear division of the vestibulocochlear (VIIIth) nerve, with an enlargement of each of the principal neuronal types. AVCN = anterior ventral cochlear nucleus; PVCN = posterior ventral cochlear nucleus; DCN = dorsal cochlear nucleus; Hi = high frequency end of tonotopic organization; Lo = low frequency end of tonotopic organization. **A.** a spherical bushy cell. **B.** a globular bushy cell. **C.** an octopus cell. **D.** a multipolar cell. **E.** a dorsal cochlear nucleus cell. A = axon; e.b. = endbulb of Held.

- Higher frequency fibers, from more basal regions of the cochlea, travel further into the cochlear nuclei before bifurcating. Their branches go to more dorsal and medial portions of the complex in a similarly systematic manner.

Thus the coding that occurs in the cochlea is replicated not once but three times—once in each of the three divisions of the cochlear nuclear complex (AVCN, PVCN, and DCN) (Figure 7–1). And as we shall see, this apparent redundancy holds a key to our ability to comprehend and analyze sounds of great complexity.

A. Anterior Ventral Cochlear Nucleus

Although there are several neuronal types in AVCN, **bushy cells** predominate. These cells are characterized by one or two thick dendrites that branch profusely and resemble a bush. In the anterior part of AVCN, the bushy cell bodies are spherical and are called **spherical bushy cells**; in the posterior AVCN, they are oval and are called **globular bushy cells** (Figure 7–1).

Ascending branches of type I spiral ganglion neurons synapse with these bushy cells as large calyceal endings called **endbulbs of Held**. Each endbulb of Held nearly surrounds the bushy cell body on which it synapses, thus creating a large synaptic area. This enables each action potential of the ascending fiber to depolarize the bushy cell sufficiently to cause an action potential in its axon. In effect, it creates a relay function (as opposed to a processing function) between the ascending branch of the nerve and the bushy cell. The physiological consequence is that the output from bushy cells maintains the precise frequency and intensity specificity, as well as the temporal relationships, that were coded in the cochlea.

Such large synapses, and neurons with purely relay functions, are rare in the nervous system.

Bushy cell axons are large and myelinated. As they exit AVCN they form the **ventral acoustic stria**—the largest tract of fibers leaving the cochlear nuclear complex. This stria enters the inferior part of the **pontine tegmentum**. As it approaches the **superior olivary complex** it gets a new name—the **trapezoid body** (Figure 7–2).

B. Posterior Ventral Cochlear Nucleus

PVCN also contains several neuronal types. **Octopus cells** predominate (Figure 7–1). They have large cell bodies with thick dendrites that extend from only one side of the cell soma and resemble the tentacles of an octopus. These dendrites course at right angles to the descending branches of spiral ganglion axons; they ramify into stubby branches only near their ends.

Both dendrites and cell bodies of octopus cells receive small terminal boutons from descending branches of many spiral ganglion central fibers. Because of this, octopus cells are most sensitive to a relatively wide band of frequencies, rather than to an extremely narrow band.

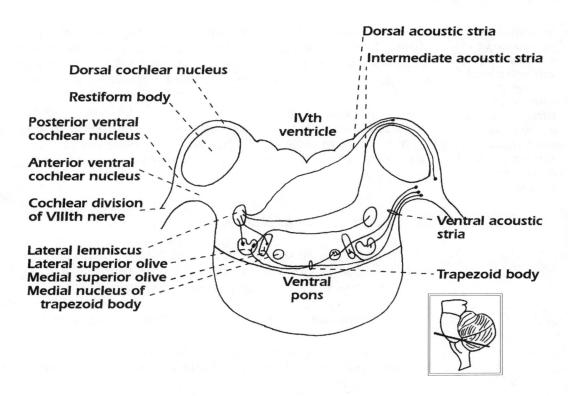

Figure 7–2. Section through the cochlear nuclear complex and superior olivary complex at the level shown in the insert. The fundamental input and output neural circuitry of the superior olivary complex is shown for information coming from the right cochlear nuclear complex. (In this and the following figures, the size of the SOC is exaggerated relative to the rest of the brainstem.)

The axons of octopus cells leave PVCN as the **intermediate acoustic stria**, also known as the **stria of Held**, which arches over the **restiform body** before entering the pontine tegmentum (Figure 7–2).

C. Multipolar Cells of AVCN and PVCN

In addition to the predominant cell types of AVCN and PVCN, there are both large and small **multipolar cells** scattered throughout VCN (Figure 7–1; box "When a Word Has Two Meanings"), and most abundantly so just caudal to the incoming nerve root. They have irregularly shaped somas from which extend several profusely branched dendrites. The dendrites are often in a stellate (star-shaped) arrangement; but sometimes, at the edge of the cochlear nuclei, they are in a parallel arrangement. These multipolar cells

Note that we pay particular attention to the initiation and ending of sounds, and little attention to continuous, unchanging sounds (such as an air conditioner).

receive bouton synaptic endings, primarily on their dendrites, from spiral ganglion axons. They respond most sensitively to the onset and termination of a sound, or to any change in the intensity or frequency of a continuing sound.

Most multipolar cell axons exit the cochlear nuclei in the ventral acoustic stria, along with bushy cell axons. A few, from multipolar cells in PVCN, leave by a more dorsal route and form a small part of the intermediate acoustic stria (stria of Held).

D. Dorsal Cochlear Nucleus

The human AVCN and PVCN are similar in their organization to those of nonhuman animals. The human DCN, by contrast, resembles only that of anthropoid apes.

In most mammals, DCN has a laminar (layered) organization:

- The outermost layer, which contains primarily axons and dendrites and very few neurons, is called the **molecular layer**.
- Just deep to it is a layer called either the **fusiform cell layer** or the **granule cell layer**. It contains many small **granule cells**: cells with a very small soma, short stubby dendrites, and a thin axon extending into the molecular layer and bifurcating there. Among the granule cells are a few **fusiform cells**, which are much larger. They have apical dendrites that extend into the molecular layer and basal dendrites that extend into the deeper layers of the nucleus.
- The deepest layer is composed of **stellate cells**. They are multipolar cells whose dendrites frequently run parallel to the surface of DCN but sometimes extend up into the granule layer and even into the molecular layer. Stellate cells are both large and small and have a complex geometry with branching dendrites on which descending branches of type I spiral ganglion cells terminate. Stellate cell axons exit DCN as the **dorsal acoustic stria (stria of Monakow)** (Figure 7–2); it courses dorsal to the restiform body and enters the pontine tegmentum just below the fourth ventricle.

In humans, there is neither a molecular layer nor a granule or fusiform layer; their cell types occur nowhere in DCN. The only neuronal cell bodies found in the human DCN are stellate cells (Figure 7–1).

WHEN A WORD HAS TWO MEANINGS

Most neurons are unipolar (having one process), bipolar (having two processes), or multipolar (having more than two—that is, an axon and at least two dendrites). Almost all neurons in the central nervous system are multipolar in this generic use of the term.

In the cochlear nuclei, for instance, each octopus cell has several processes and thus is multipolar.

Unfortunately a specific group of cells in the ventral cochlear nucleus is designated as *the* multipolar cells of AVCN and PVCN. That can be ambiguous.

But the careful student, researcher, or teacher will learn to read the meaning from the context, much as we must also do in distinguishing the nucleus of a cell from a nucleus of the brain.

1. What Is the Function of DCN?

In most mammals, DCN neurons exhibit complex physiological responses to auditory stimuli; however, destroying DCN does not appear to affect their auditory abilities. The function of DCN therefore remains a mystery in these mammals. It is even more of a mystery in humans, where its structure differs so greatly from the usual mammalian pattern (see box "The Human Dorsal Cochlear Nucleus").

Summary

The cochlear nuclear complex is divisible into the anterior ventral cochlear nucleus (AVCN), posterior ventral cochlear nucleus (PVCN), and dorsal cochlear nucleus (DCN). All three of these nuclei are tonotopically arranged. Bushy cells of the AVCN receive endbulbs of Held, are relay nuclei, and project their axons via the ventral acoustic stria. Octopus cells of the PVCN receive terminal boutons from many spiral ganglion neurons, are most sensitive to frequency bandwidths, and project their axons via the intermediate acoustic stria. Multipolar cells of the ventral cochlear nuclei receive terminal boutons from primary VIIIth nerve neurons, code for onset and termination of a sound, and project their axons via both the ventral and intermediate acoustic striae.

(continued)

THE HUMAN DORSAL COCHLEAR NUCLEUS: AN ENIGMA

We humans tend to consider our species the apex of evolution and our brain the best of all possible brains. The idea that the human brain contains a part that is less developed than in other animals is disturbing.

All species, including humans, are the products of evolution—a process driven by random mutations. When selective pressure is intense, species either become extinct or they evolve mechanisms, based on those random mutations, that enable them to adapt to the environment and survive. The more intense the pressure, the more elaborate and finely tuned the mechanisms are likely to be. When selective pressure is not intense—when any old thing will do because the species is not under threat of extinction—there is little likelihood that an elaborate mechanism will evolve.

How does that apply to what we know about the human dorsal cochlear nucleus? That would be easier to answer if we knew what this structure does in mammals where it is well developed.

What we do know:

- Human discriminations of frequency, intensity, and temporal information are as acute as those in any tested mammal.
- Human hearing is as sensitive as that of any tested mammal.
- Human high-frequency hearing is poor. High-frequency cutoff is at about 20,000 Hz; for most mammals it is up to 60,000 Hz, or even 120,000 Hz (for some bats).
- Human sound localization is less accurate than that of some other mammals (e.g., bats) and even of some birds (e.g., owls).

Since human hearing is not the "best" in all aspects, it is not surprising that parts of the human hearing apparatus are not as elaborate as those in some other mammals.

The human dorsal cochlear nucleus has a much simpler organization than that of almost all other mammals. Its stellate cells project their axons via the dorsal acoustic stria. Its functioning is unknown.

II. SUPERIOR OLIVARY COMPLEX

In the ventral inferior portion of the pontine tegmentum lies the **superior olivary complex** (SOC)—a group of small auditory nuclei that play large integrative roles in processing auditory information. They receive their synaptic input primarily from the bushy cells of AVCN, via the ventral acoustic stria and trapezoid body.

SOC contains three major nuclei: the small **lateral superior olivary nucleus**, or **lateral superior olive (LSO)**; the larger **medial superior olivary nucleus**, or **medial superior olive (MSO)**; and the very small **medial nucleus of the trapezoid body (MNTB)** (Figure 7–2). These three nuclei are surrounded by several other smaller and more diffuse nuclei, collectively called the **periolivary nuclei**.

A. Medial Superior Olivary Nucleus

MSO is the largest component of SOC in humans, as it is in most mammals with good low-frequency hearing. It is also the first place in the auditory system where what is heard in the right ear and what is heard in the left ear come together on individual neurons, allowing for **binaural interaction**.

Each principal neuron of MSO has an axon that enters the tract called the **lateral lemniscus** and two dendrites that extend from the cell body in opposite directions—one toward the right side of MSO and one toward its left side. Axons from spherical bushy cells of the right AVCN terminate as boutons on the right dendrites; axons from spherical bushy cells of the left AVCN on the left dendrites. The spherical bushy cells that synapse on the principal neurons in the MSO are located in the ventrolateral part of AVCN and thus are low-frequency neurons.

The principal neurons of MSO analyze the difference in arrival times of a sound that reaches first one ear and then the other. They propagate action potentials whose pattern is dependent on that difference. Thus they code for **sound localization** in the horizontal plane. The axons of MSO neurons extend into, and contribute to, the ipsilateral lateral lemniscus, which is a large auditory tract extending to the midbrain (Figure 7–3).

B. Medial Nucleus of the Trapezoid Body

MNTB is difficult to identify in humans, and some investigators have even suggested that it is not present. However, studies have established it as a small group of neurons in the ventral **pontine tegmentum**. Its principal neurons are multipolar. They receive input from large **calyceal endings** that resemble endbulbs of Held and come from the high frequency globular bushy cells of the contralateral AVCN.

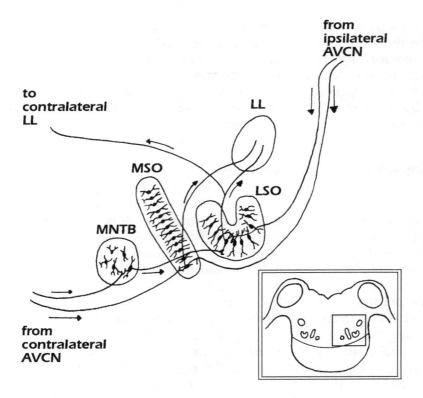

Figure 7–3. Section through right superior olivary complex as shown in lower right insert. Basic input and output circuitry of the superior olivary complex are shown. Arrows indicate directions of action potential propagation. AVCN = anterior ventral cochlear nucleus; LL = lateral lemniscus; LSO = lateral superior olive; MNTB = medial nucleus of the trapezoid body; MSO = medial superior olive.

The axons of these principal cells of MNTB terminate on the principal neurons of ipsilateral LSO (Figure 7–3).

C. Lateral Superior Olivary Nucleus

In humans, LSO is considerably smaller than MSO. Its principal neurons are also multipolar. They receive bouton-type synaptic endings from high frequency globular bushy cell axons of ipsilateral AVCN and from principal cell axons of ipsilateral MNTB (Figure 7–3). As in MSO, these connections bring information from both ears: information from the ipsilateral ear comes directly from AVCN; information from the contralateral ear comes from AVCN by way of its projection to MNTB and MNTB's projection to LSO. LSO therefore is another site of binaural integration.

LSO neurons, like those of MSO, function in horizontal sound localization. However, while MSO neurons code for time differences and thus analyze low frequencies, LSO neurons code for **intensity differences** and thus analyze high frequencies. This is explained by the difference in wave lengths. The wave lengths of low frequencies are long; they are therefore refracted around objects, such as a head, and in most head orientations will reach one ear sooner than the other. The wave lengths of high frequencies are equal to or shorter than the dimensions of the head and therefore reflect off the head. This creates a partial "sound shadow" at the ear opposite the sound source, which makes the sound more intense at the ear nearer the source than at the opposite ear.

If this is confusing, think of this analogy: High frequencies are like light rays, which have very short wave lengths. They reflect off surfaces; they do not go around corners but create shadows instead. Low frequencies, like water, pass around (are refracted by) obstacles such as rocks in a stream.

The axons of LSO neurons contribute bilaterally to the lateral lemnisci (Figure 7–3), which carry information to the midbrain.

Thus a major function of the superior olivary complex is to code for auditory localization in the horizontal plane (see box "Variations in the Superior Olivary Complex"). However, the *perception* of localization occurs not here but, milliseconds later, in the **cerebral cortex** where consciousness exists.

D. Stapedius Reflex

Some axons from both LSO and MSO synapse bilaterally with a small group of neurons of the **facial nucleus**, which also lies in the pontine tegmentum. From there, axons extend out of the brainstem, as part of the **VIIth cranial (facial) nerve**, to innervate the **stapedius muscle** of the middle ear. As discussed in Chapter 6, the stapedius muscle contracts reflexively in response to intense sounds. Part of its reflex arc involves the superior olivary complex; the connection from sensory input to motor output occurs between the superior olivary complex and the facial nucleus (Figure 7–4).

The neurons of the facial nucleus that innervate the stapedius muscle are a distinct group, which lies just outside the rest of the facial nucleus.

VARIATIONS IN THE SUPERIOR OLIVARY COMPLEX

There is more variation among the three major components of the mammalian SOC than in any other central auditory structure.

- In low-frequency hearers, such as humans, MSO is far larger than LSO and MNTB.
- In high-frequency hearers with poor low-frequency hearing, such as bats, mice, and whales, LSO and MNTB are large and MSO is sometimes so small that it is difficult to identify.
- In mammals with sensitive hearing across a broad frequency spectrum, such as cats and guinea pigs, MSO, LSO, and MNTB are all prominent.

So precise are these correlations that a fairly accurate estimate of an animal's frequency range can be based on the relative sizes of these three SOC components.

A major function of these nuclei is coding for sound localization in horizontal space. MSO codes low frequencies, using differences in their arrival times at each ear. LSO and MNTB code high frequencies, using differences in intensity at each ear.

Such an elaborate scheme of structure and variation to accomplish a function suggests that knowing a sound's source is nearly as important as detecting the sound in the first place. Whether it means danger, food, or sex, the second thing an animal needs to know about a sound is *where is it?* Thus it is not surprising that the structures that evolved to answer that question are prominent and finely correlated with their functional abilities.

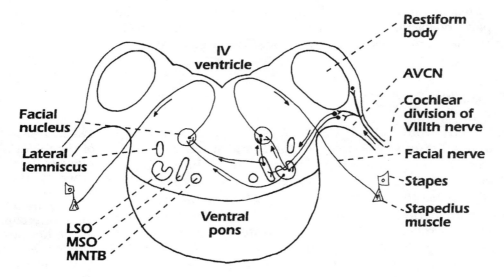

Figure 7–4. Coronal section of brainstem showing the basic neural circuitry of the stapedius reflex. AVCN = anterior ventral cochlear nucleus; LSO = lateral superior olive; MSO = medial superior olivary nucleus; MNTB = medial nucleus of the trapezoid body.

E. Periolivary Nuclei

The best understood groups of neurons in the periolivary nuclei are those whose axons form the **olivocochlear bundle**. They are readily divided into a medial group and a lateral group (Figure 7–5).

The medial group, or **medial olivocochlear bundle**, is made up of large multipolar neurons. Although some of their axons travel to the ipsilateral cochlea, most cross the midline and leave the brain as part of the contralateral **vestibular division of the vestibulocochlear nerve**. Then, by way of the **anastomosis of Oort**, they enter the cochlea. There they spiral within **Rosenthal's canal** as the **intraganglionic spiral bundle** before passing out to the organ of Corti and terminating as large vesiculated synapses on **outer hair cells**.

Rosenthal's canal is the bony channel within the modiolus that contains the spiral ganglion.

The lateral group, or **lateral olivocochlear bundle**, is made up of smaller multipolar neurons, joined perhaps by some multipolar neurons of LSO. These neurons send most of their axons ipsilaterally (although some travel to the contralateral cochlea). These axons also leave the brain as part of the vestibular division of the vestibulocochlear nerve. They follow the anastomosis of Oort, enter the cochlea, and form part of the intraganglionic spiral bundle.

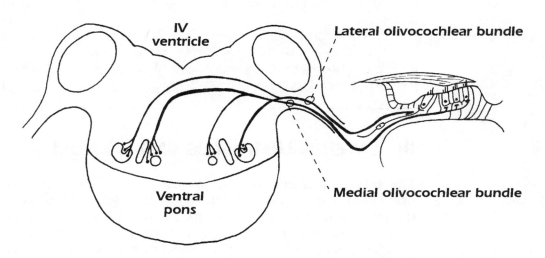

Figure 7–5. Organization of the olivocochlear bundles projecting to the right organ of Corti.

While neurons of the medial olivocochlear bundle end on **outer hair cells**, those of the lateral olivocochlear bundle terminate as small vesiculated endings on the **peripheral processes of type I spiral ganglion neurons** just below the inner hair cells. As described in Chapter 6, the information that the olivocochlear bundle carries back to the cochlea enables the brain to modulate the sensitivity of, and activity within, the cochlea.

Summary

The superior olivary complex (SOC) lies in the ventral pontine tegmentum. The medial superior olivary nucleus (MSO) receives input from spherical bushy neurons of both right and left AVCN nuclei. Because of this binaural input, MSO neurons code for low frequency horizontal sound localization by comparing the times of arrival of sounds from the right and left ears.

The lateral superior olivary nucleus (LSO) codes for high frequency horizontal sound localization by comparing sound intensity from the right and left ears. LSO neurons receive input directly from ipsilateral globular bushy cells and, indirectly—via synapses in the medial nucleus of the trapezoid body—from the contralateral bushy cells.

Both MSO and LSO project their axons via the lateral lemniscus.

The SOC is also an integral portion of the stapedius reflex. The cell bodies of the olivocochlear bundle are part of the SOC's periolivary nuclei .

III. LATERAL LEMNISCUS AND ITS NUCLEI

The **lateral lemniscus**, the largest tract of the auditory brainstem, carries information to the **inferior colliculus** in the midbrain. Although named as one tract, it is actually six distinct pathways that are both structurally and functionally parallel. They are formed just lateral to the superior olivary complex by the axons of six different cell groups, which enter the lateral lemniscus via different routes (Figure 7–6):

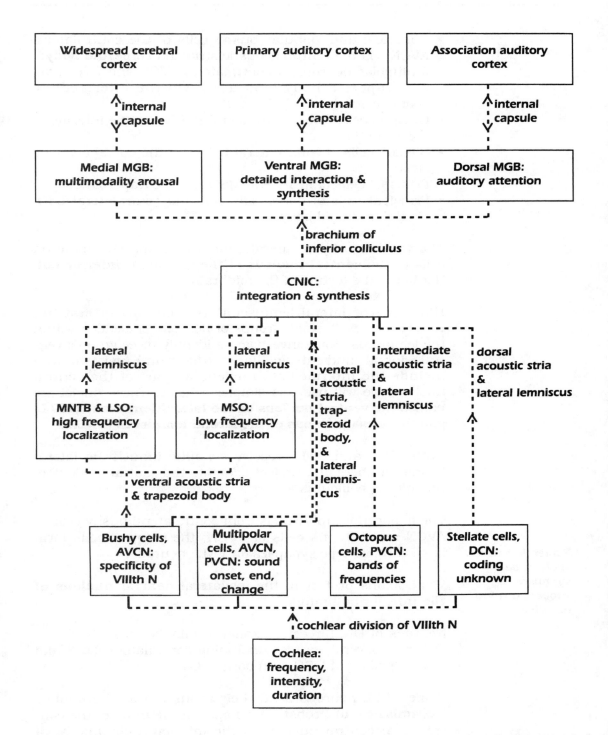

Figure 7–6. Block diagram of the central auditory pathways, illustrating divergence of information to the cochlear nuclear complex, establishment of parallel pathways, convergence to the central nucleus of the inferior colliculus, and then another divergence to the medial geniculate body and cerebral cortex.

- Spherical and globular bushy cells of the contralateral AVCN, via the ventral acoustic stria and **trapezoid body**;
- Multipolar neurons of contralateral AVCN and PVCN, via the trapezoid body (and a few via the intermediate acoustic stria);
- Octopus cells from contralateral PVCN, via the intermediate acoustic stria;
- Stellate cells of contralateral DCN, via the dorsal acoustic stria;
- Principal cells of ipsilateral MSO, via the trapezoid body;
- Principal cells of both ipsilateral and contralateral LSO, via the trapezoid body.

The vast majority of lateral lemniscal axons terminate on cells of the **central nucleus** of the ipsilateral **inferior colliculus** in the tectum of the midbrain.

However, the lateral lemniscus also contains **interstitial nuclei**—relatively small groups of neurons embedded within the lemniscus. Some investigators identify three groups: ventral, dorsal, and intermediate. Others find just two, and include the intermediate nucleus as part of the ventral nucleus; we will use this simpler scheme. These nuclei are named the **ventral nucleus of the lateral lemniscus (VNLL)** and the **dorsal nucleus of the lateral lemniscus (DNLL)**.

Both VNLL and DNLL receive synaptic input from lateral lemniscal fibers and project axons to the central nucleus of the inferior colliculus.

The major input to VNLL is from contralateral bushy cells of AVCN and octopus cells of PVCN; the octopus cells form large calyceal-type synapses on VNLL neurons.

Remember that such large synapses suggest a relay function.

VNLL axons project to the ipsilateral **central nucleus of the inferior colliculus**.

Neurons of DNLL receive axonal terminals (mostly collaterals) from several sources, including contralateral DCN and AVCN, ipsilateral MSO, and both LSOs.

Some DNLL neurons send their axons across the midline (**commissure of Probst**) to synapse on neurons of the contralateral central nucleus of the inferior colliculus. Most DNLL neurons project, via the lateral lemniscus, to the ipsilateral central nucleus of the inferior colliculus.

Summary

The lateral lemniscus contains axons from several auditory nuclei traveling in parallel: bushy cells of AVCN, octopus cells of PVCN, multipolar cells of VCN, stellate cells of DCN, principal cells of MSO, and principal cells of LSO. There are two nuclei in the lateral lemniscus—the dorsal nucleus of the lateral lemniscus (DNLL) and the ventral nucleus of the lateral lemniscus (VNLL). Axons of the lateral lemniscus project to the central nucleus of the inferior colliculus (CNIC).

IV. INFERIOR COLLICULUS

Finally we reach the largest midbrain auditory center: the **inferior colliculus**. Its dominant feature is the **central nucleus of the inferior colliculus (CNIC)**.

The principal and most numerous neurons of CNIC are small, multipolar **fusiform cells** whose dendrites are oriented in oblique, parallel laminae. These dendrites, which end in small "tufted" branchings, are called **bitufted** (Figure 7–7). The laminae maintain the tonotopic organization first established in the cochlea.

The fusiform cells receive their synaptic input from the lateral lemniscus and the commissure of Probst.

A few of their axons course across the midline as the **commissure of the inferior colliculus** (Figure 7–7); they then synapse on principal cells in contralateral CNIC, or continue through CNIC to form part of the contralateral **brachium of the inferior colliculus**. However, most principal cell axons form the brachium of the ipsilateral inferior colliculus, which lies on the dorsolateral surface of the inferior colliculus (Figure 7–7). The brachium of the inferior colliculus extends out of the brainstem and synapses on thalamic auditory nuclei that make up the **medial geniculate body (MGB)**.

In addition to CNIC, the inferior colliculus has two smaller nuclei. On the dorsal and posterior surfaces is its **pericen-**

Before it reaches the commissure of the inferior colliculus, auditory information has already crossed from the side of entry to the opposite side several times. Most (but not all) of what is heard in one ear is interpreted by the opposite cerebral hemisphere.

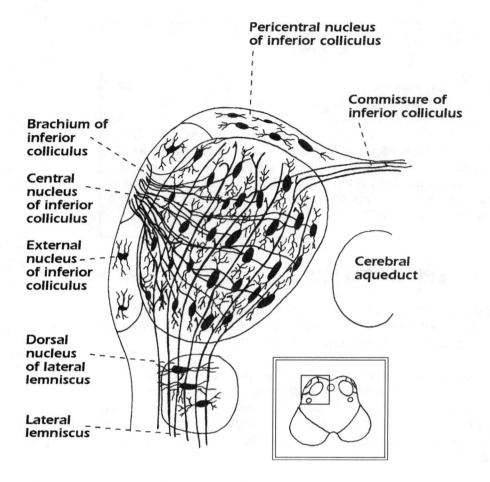

Figure 7-7. Coronal section through the left inferior colliculus showing neural circuitry and neuronal organization. Lower right insert is for orientation.

tral nucleus; on the lateral surface, its **external nucleus** (Figure 7-7). The pericentral nucleus has a layered structure reminiscent of a cortex. It receives axonal input from CNIC and descending projections from auditory cortex; it projects axons to MGB. The external nucleus is composed of heterogeneous neuronal types with no single type predominating. It receives axonal input from CNIC and from collaterals of ascending somesthetic axons. It projects its axons, via the brachium of the inferior colliculus, to the medial geniculate body.

Summary

The central nucleus of the inferior colliculus (CNIC) is the largest brainstem auditory nucleus. It receives most of its input from the lateral lemniscus and projects axons via the brachium of the inferior colliculus to the medial geniculate body (MGB). Its fusiform principal neurons are bitufted and arranged in tonotopic laminae. The inferior colliculus also contains a pericentral nucleus and an external nucleus.

V. ORGANIZATION OF AUDITORY BRAINSTEM: OVERVIEW

We have noted that, through a series of anatomical structures and their correlated physiological events, auditory information from the cochlea is replicated as soon as it enters the cochlear nuclear complex and is arranged in three separate tonotopic groupings. Each of these groupings belongs to a different pathway; each pathway carries different information to the midbrain (Figure 7–6; box "Auditory Brainstem Pathways").

- In AVCN, bushy cells are sharply tuned and maintain the frequency, intensity, and temporal coding established in the cochlea; bushy cell axons carry much of that information to the superior olivary complex. However, some bushy cell axons bypass the superior olivary complex and travel directly to the contralateral CNIC via the lateral lemniscus.
- In PVCN, octopus cells are tuned more broadly than the primary neurons and are therefore most responsive to broad bands rather than to very narrow bands of frequencies.
- In DCN, although some complex coding occurs in nonhuman mammals, the situation in humans is unclear. Certainly they carry information, but what it is continues to elude us.

These pathways are three of six separate pathways from the ear to the midbrain outlined in the overview of the lateral lemniscus (Section III above).

A fourth, parallel pathway originates in the cochlear nuclei from axons of multipolar neurons throughout PVCN and AVCN that are very sensitive to the onset and termination of sounds. This pathway carries this information—via the ventral acoustic stria, trapezoid body, and to some extent intermediate acoustic stria—to the contralateral lateral lemniscus, and from there to the inferior colliculus.

Two additional pathways carry information from the superior olivary complex to the CNIC (Figure 7-6).

- From neurons of LSO, axons project bilaterally in the lateral lemniscus and carry high frequency, horizontal sound localization information to the CNIC.
- From neurons of MSO, axons project ipsilaterally in the lateral lemniscus and carry low frequency, horizontal sound localization information to the CNIC.

There are two other brainstem auditory pathways, for a total of eight: the olivocochlear bundle, and the stapedius reflex. These two pathways direct auditory information back to the auditory periphery. Meanwhile, the six parallel ascending pathways go their separate ways, only to converge upon CNIC, whose neuropil represents, as far as we know, a single tonotopic arrangement.

We may ask if this is needlessly complicated; after all, if it is all going to come together in the upper brainstem anyway, what purpose is served by having six separate ascending pathways through the lower brainstem?

The answer is elegant: In each of the six divergent, yet parallel, pathways, auditory information is processed (coded) for different attributes (frequency specificity, frequency bands, time of onset, etc.); thus each pathway requires its own neural network. However, in order for all these separate pieces of the code to be recognized as aspects of the same acoustic stimulus, they must finally be brought back together again. This is what happens in the CNIC.

Now we can see that the auditory brainstem is not only a series of relay stations but, more importantly, a network of separate, interwoven neuronal mechanisms, exquisitely adapted to code and transmit highly specific, detailed information from the auditory periphery to the midbrain.

AUDITORY BRAINSTEM PATHWAYS ARE UNIQUE

Parallel ascending pathways are a common characteristic in systems that process neural information.

Visual System

- A major pathway goes from retina to lateral geniculate body (thalamus), then to visual cortex.
- A parallel pathway goes from retina to superior colliculus, then to thalamus and visual cortex.

Somesthetic System (Touch, Pain, Temperature, Pressure)

- A major pathway, the dorsal column system, goes from the dorsal roots of spinal nerves directly to the nuclei gracilis and cuneatus in the lower brainstem, then to the ventral posterior lateral nucleus of the thalamus, and finally to the somesthetic cortex. This system codes for fine discriminative touch, proprioception, and pressure.
- A parallel spinothalamic system goes from the dorsal roots and synapses on cells in the spinal cord, then to posterior ventrolateral thalamus, then to somesthetic cortex.

Voluntary Motor System

- A major pathway goes from motor cortex, to ventral horn cells of the spinal cord, to skeletal muscles.
- A parallel pathway goes from motor cortex to the red nucleus in the tegmentum of the midbrain, to the ventral horn of the spinal cord, to skeletal muscles.

How is the Auditory System Different?

As you see, parallel pathways are the norm rather than the exception. The brainstem auditory system, however, is unique in three ways:

- It has more parallel pathways than other systems.
- They synapse on more brainstem nuclei.
- They converge in the midbrain and then diverge again—going to the medial geniculate body, the thalamic auditory center—and finally to the auditory cortex.

The earliest vertebrates undoubtedly had serviceable tactile, visual, and motor systems, but they were probably deaf. Hearing evolved independently in many groups of later vertebrates: in several groups of fishes, in many amphibians, in the group of reptiles that gave rise to today's reptiles and birds, and in the group of reptiles that gave rise to mammals.

Evolutionarily speaking, the mammalian auditory system is the new kid on the block. It is not surprising that its processing system is not fully analogous to that of other systems.

Summary

Six functionally distinct groups of axons, each coded for different aspects of sound stimuli, travel in the lateral lemniscus to synapse on a single tonotopically organized nucleus—the central nucleus of the inferior colliculus (CNIC). In this way, the diverse aspects of the sound signal are synthesized into a whole before being transmitted to the auditory forebrain.

VI. AUDITORY BRAINSTEM RESPONSES

In the clinic it is possible to test the integrity of the auditory portions of a person's brainstem by recording **auditory brainstem responses** (**ABRs**). In this procedure, surface electrodes are placed on the person's skin over each mastoid (just behind the ear) and on the vertex (top of the head). These electrodes are wired to an amplifier, a computer, a chart recorder, and a video screen. Repetitive brief tone bursts or clicks are then presented. These brief stimuli evoke synchronous action potentials in a large number of VIIIth nerve central fibers; these synchronous action potentials, in turn, cause synchronous activity of neurons in the cochlear nuclear complex, superior olivary complex, lateral lemnisci, and inferior colliculi. At each of these synapses, there is an extremely brief delay while neurotransmitters are released and depolarization occurs.

Wave I originates in the VIIIth nerve near the cochlea. Wave II originates from the VIIIth nerve and adjacent cochlear nuclei. Waves III–V have multiple origins, from the superior olive to the inferior colliculus.

The synchronous firing of many neurons produces an electrical potential large enough to be detected by the electrodes on the skin. The computer filters out all electrical events that are not synchronized with the rate of tone bursts or clicks (the "noise"), and the amplifier amplifies what remains (the "signal"). The result is a recording of the auditory brainstem response, or ABR—the electrical potentials produced by the auditory neurons in the VIIIth nerve and the brainstem in response to brief auditory stimuli. The ABR is comprised of **five major potentials**—called **waves**, because they appear on the recorder and video screen as humps or waves. One can measure how large each wave is (its **amplitude**), and how many milliseconds after the stimulus it appears (its **latency**). These amplitudes and latencies can then be compared with those of people with known normal hearing.

By this method, hearing can be objectively evaluated even in an infant or in someone, say, in a coma, who is unable to cooperate with a subjective test ("hold up your hand when you hear the sound"). Obviously an abnormal ABR can be due to a middle ear or cochlear problem as well as to a brainstem problem. Therefore if an abnormal ABR is found, further testing is necessary. However, a normal ABR is a strong indicator that the middle ear, cochlea, and auditory brainstem are all functioning normally.

Summary

Auditory brainstem responses (ABRs) are the summed responses of the synchronous firing of large numbers of VIIIth nerve and auditory brainstem neurons. By measuring the amplitude and latencies of each of the five major waves of the auditory brainstem response, one can objectively evaluate the hearing of people who are unable to report their perceptions—including infants and people with acute or chronic handicaps.

VII. AUDITORY FOREBRAIN

The **forebrain** includes both the **diencephalon** and the **cerebral hemispheres**. The auditory portion of the diencephalon is the **medial geniculate body (MGB)** of the thalamus. This complex nuclear group is divided into a **ventral division**, a **dorsal division**, and a **medial division** (Figure 7–8). Auditory information is brought to MGB by the brachium of the inferior colliculus, a tract formed by axons whose cell bodies are in the inferior colliculus.

Most fibers of the brachium of the inferior colliculus terminate in the ventral division of MGB. Like other auditory nuclei, it is **tonotopically organized**, with parallel laminae of **bitufted neurons** much like the principal neurons of CNIC. It receives detailed auditory information, including precise information about the source and location, onset and offset, and frequency and intensity of a sound. Its axons further process this information and then project it via the **sublenticular portion of the internal capsule to primary auditory cortex**. The ventral division of MGB also

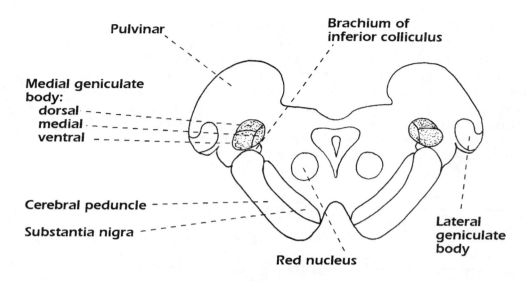

Figure 7–8. Coronal section through the junction of the diencephalon and midbrain showing the position of the medial geniculate body and its divisions.

"Sublenticular" refers to the portion of the internal capsule ventral to the lenticular nucleus.

receives many axons from primary auditory cortex. (It is a general characteristic of thalamo-cortical projections that there is always a reciprocal cortico-thalamic projection—from the cortex back to a thalamic nucleus.)

The other two divisions of MGB—the dorsal and the medial divisions—receive less specific auditory information than does the ventral division. However, fibers of the brachium of the inferior colliculus project to both of these divisions.

The dorsal division of MGB contains neurons of several morphological types and is tonotopically organized. It has reciprocal interconnections with the ventral division. The neurons of the dorsal division project axons primarily to **association auditory cortices** by way of the internal capsule. It has been proposed that the dorsal division functions in maintaining and directing **auditory attention**.

The medial division of MGB is composed of large multipolar neurons that are not as tightly packed together as are the neurons in the ventral and dorsal divisions. In addition to axons from the brachium of the inferior colliculus, the medial division also receives **vestibular, somesthetic,** and **visual information**. Thus the medial division is a multimodal nucleus of the thalamus, not a purely auditory division of MGB. The axons from the medial division project diffusely to both auditory and nonauditory cortices and to the

basal ganglia, particularly the **putamen** and the **amygdala**. All cortical regions, both auditory and nonauditory, also send some projections to the medial division of MGB via the internal capsule. It has been proposed that the medial division functions as a multi-sensory **arousal system**, essentially telling the brain to pay attention to what is going on.

This arousal function is similar to one of the functions of the reticular formation.

In summary, MGB receives its major input from the inferior colliculus via the brachium of the inferior colliculus. The MGB's ventral division—its most specific auditory division—both processes and relays specific detailed auditory information to the primary auditory cortex. Its dorsal division, which receives less specific auditory information, is an auditory attention nucleus; its major projection is to association auditory cortices. The medial division receives multimodal input and projects diffusely to both cortical and non-cortical areas of the forebrain.

Thus the convergence of auditory information in CNIC is followed by another divergence. The largest pathway in this new divergence carries specific auditory information to the ventral division of MGB and then to primary auditory cortex. A second pathway goes to the dorsal division of MGB for auditory attention. A third pathway travels in the brachium of the inferior colliculus to the medial division of MGB, where it contributes to a multimodal general arousal function and then directs this general arousal to cerebral cortex and basal ganglia.

Auditory information from all three divisions leaves MGB via the **sublenticular portion of the internal capsule** (Figure 7–9), and then enters cerebral cortex. There, on the superior surface of the temporal lobe but visible only if one separates the edges of the **Sylvian fissure** and looks deeply within (Figure 7–10), are from one to three **transverse gyri of Heschl**, which contain the primary auditory cortices (**Brodmann's areas 41 and 42**). The number of gyri varies not only from brain to brain but also from side to side in the same brain. Details of the auditory cortices will be discussed in Chapter 8.

There is no sharp boundary marking where auditory projections and auditory processing end and decoding for speech and language begin. Much of the information we need for decoding speech is actually processed—that is, decoded—in subcortical auditory nuclei. However, all indications are that conscious speech processing occurs at cortical levels. This is the subject of Section III of this book, which examines speech and language.

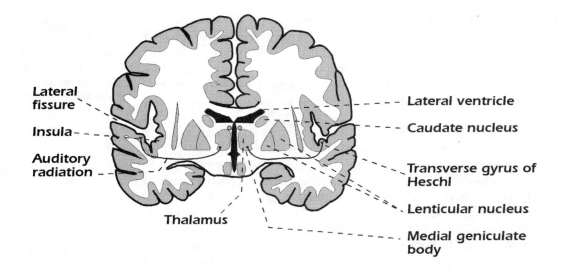

Figure 7–9. Coronal section through the medial geniculate body showing the projection of axons through the sublenticular portion of the internal capsule to the transverse gyri of Heschl.

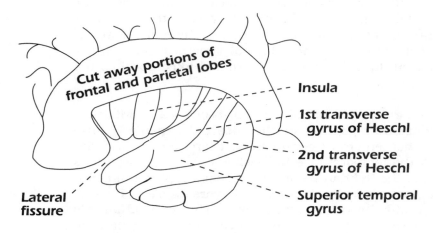

Figure 7–10. Diagram of the left cerebral hemisphere with parts of the frontal and parietal lobes above the lateral fissure cut away. This allows visualization of the insula and transverse gyri of Heschl.

Summary

The forebrain is the diencephalon and cerebrum. The auditory portion of the diencephalon is the medial geniculate body (MGB) of the thalamus. The ventral division of MGB is composed of tonotopically arranged laminae of bitufted principal neurons. It processes detailed auditory information and projects its axons via the sublenticular portion of the internal capsule to the primary auditory cortices of the transverse gyri of Heschl. The dorsal division of MGB receives both from the ventral division and from the inferior colliculus. It projects auditory attention information to association auditory cortices. The medial division of MGB is a multimodal nucleus that projects nonspecific arousal information diffusely to the cerebral cortex and basal ganglia.

CHAPTER 7 SUMMARY

Central processes of spiral ganglion neurons bifurcate in the cochlear nuclear complex into ascending and descending branches, all of which are tonotopically organized. The ascending branches go to the anterior ventral cochlear nucleus (AVCN); the descending branches go first to the posterior ventral cochlear nucleus (PVCN) and then to the dorsal cochlear nucleus (DCN).

Bushy cells of AVCN receive large synapses, called endbulbs of Held; these cells act as relay neurons. Their axons form most of the ventral acoustic stria. Octopus cells of PVCN code for frequency bandwidth; their axons form most of the intermediate acoustic stria. Multipolar cells of the ventral cochlear nuclei code for onset and termination of stimuli; their axons contribute to the ventral and intermediate acoustic striae. The human DCN is less elaborate than that of most mammals. Its axons form the dorsal acoustic stria. The function of this nucleus remains obscure.

The superior olivary complex (SOC) is in the ventral pontine tegmentum. The medial superior olivary nucleus (MSO) receives binaural input from spherical bushy cells, codes for low frequency horizontal sound localization from temporal cues, and projects its axons via the lateral lemniscus. The lateral superior olivary nucleus (LSO) receives information directly from ipsilateral globular bushy cells and, indirectly—via synapses in the medial nucleus of the trapezoid body (MNTB)—from contralateral globular bushy cells. It codes for high frequency horizontal sound localization from intensity cues and projects its axons via the lateral lemniscus. The SOC also participates in the stapedius reflex, and its periolivary nuclei contain the cell bodies of the olivocochlear bundle.

The lateral lemniscus contains several functionally distinct groups of axons: bushy cell axons from AVCN, octopus cell axons from PVCN, multipolar cell axons from VCN, stellate cell axons from DCN, principal cell axons from MSO, and principal cell axons from LSO. The lateral lemniscus also has two interstitial nuclei—the dorsal and ventral nuclei of the lateral lemniscus (DNLL, VNLL).

Lateral lemnisci axons terminate in the central nucleus of the inferior colliculus (CNIC), which is tonotopically arranged and integrates the diverse information brought to it by the lateral lemniscus. The bitufted principal cells of CNIC project their axons to MGB via the brachium of the inferior colliculus. The inferior colliculus also contains a pericentral nucleus and an external nucleus.

The lower nuclei of the auditory brainstem (cochlear nuclear complex, superior olivary complex, and the nuclei of the lateral lemniscus) code for different aspects of auditory stimuli and send the processed information through parallel pathways to CNIC. There, the diversely processed information is integrated and synthesized before being passed on to the auditory forebrain.

The activity of the cochlear division of the vestibulocochlear nerve and of the auditory brainstem can be monitored noninvasively, using auditory brainstem responses (ABRs).

The auditory forebrain is composed of the medial geniculate body (MGB) and auditory cortices. The ventral division of MGB does the detailed auditory processing and projects its axons via the sublenticular internal capsule to the primary auditory cortices in the transverse gyri of Heschl. The dorsal division of MGB functions for auditory attention and projects its axons to association auditory cortices. The medial division of MGB is multimodal, functions for general arousal, and projects its axons diffusely to wide areas of the cerebral cortex and to parts of the basal ganglia.

ADDITIONAL READING

Masterton, R. B. (1992). Role of the central auditory system in hearing: The new direction. *Trends in Neurosciences, 15*, 280–285.

Masterton, R. B. (1993). Central auditory system. *Otorhinolaryngology, 55*, 159–163.

Popper, A. N., & Fay, R. R. (Eds.). (1992). *The mammalian auditory pathway: Neurophysiology*. New York: Springer-Verlag.

Webster, D. B., Popper, A. N., & Fay, R. R. (Eds.). (1992). *The mammalian auditory pathway: Neuroanatomy*. New York: Springer-Verlag.

STUDY GUIDE

Answer each question with a brief paragraph

1. Describe the nuclei of the cochlear nuclear complex.

2. Describe the anatomy and physiology of octopus cells.

3. In what way is the human dorsal cochlear nucleus unusual?

4. Compare binaural processing in the medial superior olivary nucleus and binaural processing in the lateral superior olivary nucleus.

5. Describe the anatomical substrate of the stapedius reflex.

6. What are the six cell groups that contribute axons to the lateral lemniscus?

7. Describe the organization of the inferior colliculus.

8. What is the functional significance of six parallel pathways converging onto the central nucleus of the inferior colliculus?

9. What are auditory brainstem responses?

10. Describe the functional roles of the three divisions of the medial geniculate body.

11. What is the sublenticular portion of the internal capsule?

Odd One Out

In each of the following questions, choose the item that does not "fit" with the other three; briefly explain what the other three have in common that the odd one lacks. There may be more than one correct answer.

1. ___ bushy cell

   ___ multipolar cell of VCN

   ___ octopus cell

   ___ stellate cell of DCN

   WHY?

2. ___ stria vascularis

   ___ dorsal acoustic stria

   ___ intermediate acoustic stria

   ___ ventral acoustic stria

   WHY?

3. ___ dorsal nucleus of the lateral lemniscus

   ___ medial nucleus of the trapezoid body

   ___ lateral superior olivary nucleus

   ___ medial superior olivary nucleus

   WHY?

4. ___ trapezoid body

   ___ medial geniculate body

   ___ lateral geniculate body

   ___ brachium of the inferior colliculus

WHY?

5. ___ central nucleus of the inferior colliculus

   ___ medial geniculate body

   ___ ventral nucleus of the lateral lemniscus

   ___ trapezoid body

WHY?

6. ___ commissure of Probst

   ___ dorsal acoustic stria

   ___ lateral lemniscus

   ___ trapezoid body

WHY?

7. ___ sublenticular portion of the internal capsule

   ___ central nucleus of the inferior colliculus

   ___ medial geniculate body

   ___ transverse gyri of Heschl

WHY?

SECTION III
Speech and Language

Now that you understand the sensory input from the auditory (and vestibular) systems, it is time to move on to the essence of communication: speech, its major output, and language, its central integrator. Their neural organizations are extremely complex and, therefore, provide fascinating challenges to students, teachers, and researchers alike.

In this three chapter section you will learn about:

- the organization of cerebral cortex and mechanisms of speech perception (Chapter 8);
- the organization of language and how it interacts with emotions, memories, and decision making (Chapter 9);
- the organization of the nervous system in the motor act of producing speech (Chapter 10).

8

CORTICAL ORGANIZATION AND SPEECH RECEPTION

If there is a single locus of consciousness, it is the **cerebral cortex**, where our individuality and ability to think also reside.

All mammals have a cerebral cortex, with similar cellular structure and neuronal connections. However, the cerebral cortex is more extensive in humans than in all other mammals except whales and dolphins (in which it is even more extensive than in humans). It contains our faculties for speech and language, without which we would not be capable of conceptual thought. It is these capabilities, more than any others, that make us unique among animals.

Many small mammals such as mice and rats have a smooth, nonconvoluted cerebral cortex.

The cerebral cortex is made up of the gray matter that lies on the surface of the **cerebral hemispheres**. In humans, it is highly convoluted; that is, it is not a flat layer but is arranged in a series of bulges, called gyri, that alternate with grooves, called sulci, or, if extraordinarily deep, fissures. Its total area is about 2200 square centimeters (about 2.5 square feet). Its thickness varies from 4.5 millimeters (mm) in the prefrontal cortices to a mere 1.5 mm in the visual cortex of the occipital lobe. It has been estimated to contain about 14 billion neurons.

The auditory radiation is part of the sublenticular portion of the internal capsule.

Auditory information reaches the cerebral cortex from the **medial geniculate body** via a portion of the **internal capsule** called the **auditory radiation**. Some of that information is speech. Before it can be comprehended, the cerebral cortex must analyze the neural messages it receives and compare them with the memory of speech sounds.

To begin to understand these complex functions, we need to know the structural and functional organization of the cerebral cortex.

I. ORGANIZATION OF CEREBRAL CORTEX

Humans have more neocortex relative to allocortex than other mammals.

Approximately 90% of the cerebral cortex is **neocortex**, which is defined as a cerebral cortex having six distinct layers of cells. The other 10% or so is **allocortex**—a phylogenetically older cortex having just three layers. Allocortex is found in reptiles, birds, and amphibians, as well as mammals. There are a few areas of allocortex in humans, including **hippocampus**, **septal region**, **cingulate gyrus**, and **parahippocampal gyrus**. Neocortex is found only in mammals. We will focus on neocortex here.

In the early 20th century, Korbinian Brodmann published a detailed microscopic study of the human cerebral cortex. He divided it into 47 areas, based on differences in the structure of the cortical layers in each area. More recent work has shown that those structurally different areas are also functionally different, and his numbering system is still used. Although we will not explore all 47 areas, some are of particular interest to audiologists and speech-language professionals (Figure 8–1).

- **Area 4**, the **precentral gyrus**, is a **primary motor cortex**.
- **Areas 3, 1, and 2** are **primary somatosensory cortices**; they lie behind area 4, on the **postcentral gyrus** of the **parietal lobe**.
- **Area 6**, the **premotor area**, lies just in front of area 4. *and operculum!*
- **Areas 44 and 45** are the **area triangularis** in the **inferior frontal gyrus**. On one side, almost always the left, areas 44 and 45 function in expressive speech and are called **Broca's area**.
- **Areas 41 and 42** are the **transverse gyri of Heschl**, of which there may be one, two, or three per side; the number, which varies from side to side and brain to brain, has no apparent functional significance. These gyri lie on the superior surface of the **temporal lobe** and are seen only if one spreads opens the **Sylvian fissure** and looks deep within it.
- **Area 22** lies posteriorly and inferiorly to the transverse gyri of Heschl and is composed of the **planum temporale** and the adjoining **posterior two-thirds of the superior temporal** gyrus. On one side, almost always the left, area 22 functions in speech reception and is called **Wernicke's area**.
- **Area 39**, the **angular gyrus**, and **area 40**, the **supramarginal gyrus**, are located in the **inferior parietal lobule** and are important association cortices.
- **Area 17**, the **primary visual cortex**, is on gyri both above and below the **calcarine fissure** on the medial surface of the **occipital lobe**.
- **Areas 18 and 19**, association visual cortices, comprise the remainder of the occipital lobe.

A. Cell Types of Neocortex

One might expect that the complex functions of the neocortex would require many different cell types. Surprisingly, most of the neurons of the neocortex are either **pyramidal cells** or **stellate (granular) cells** (Figure 8–2).

The complex functions of neocortex result more from the number and complexity of their synaptic relationships than from the diversity of their cell types.

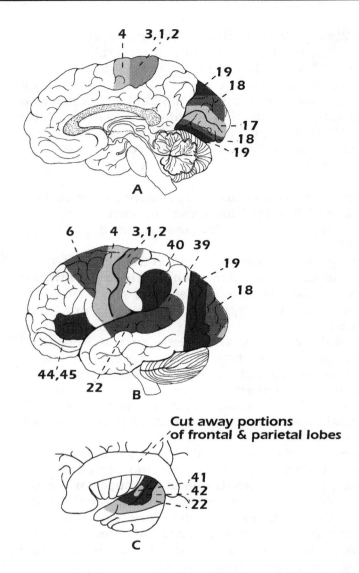

Figure 8–1. Three diagrams showing the locations of the Brodmann's areas described in the text. **A** is a medial view of the right half of the brain. **B** is a lateral view of the brain. **C** is a view of the superior surface of the left temporal lobe after removal of parts of the frontal and parietal lobes. 3, 1, and 2 = primary somesthetic cortex; 4 = primary motor cortex; 6 = premotor cortex; 17 = primary visual cortex; 18 and 19 = visual association cortex; 22 = superior temporal gyrus and planum temporale; 39 = angular gyrus; 40 = supramarginal gyrus; 41 and 42 = primary auditory cortices; 44, 45 = area triangularis.

Pyramidal cells are so named because their cell bodies are shaped roughly like pyramids. The apex always points toward the surface of the neocortex and bears a long, branched, **apical dendrite** that extends toward the pial surface. This apical dendrite has many branches that are

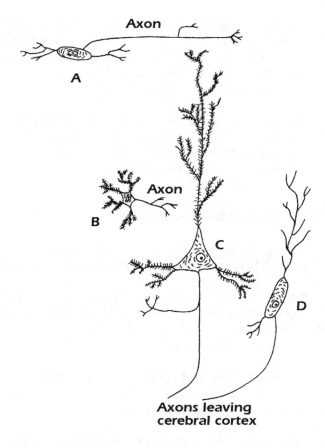

Figure 8-2. Major cell types of the neocortex. **A** is a horizontal cell of Cajal; **B** is a stellate cell; **C** is a pyramidal cell; and **D** is a fusiform cell. Note the dendritic spines on the stellate and pyramidal cells.

studded with small spines. (Spines are very short branches of dendrites that increase the surface area to allow for more synapses.) Shorter, **basal dendrites** extend from the two lower corners of the cell body; they are also branched and have many spines.

Dendritic spines are found most frequently—but not exclusively—on cortical neurons.

Stellate, or granular, cells are smaller, multipolar neurons. Although they have a less extensive dendritic arbor than the pyramidal cells, each stellate cell sends many dendrites into the area immediately surrounding its cell body. Some of these branched dendrites bear spines; others do not.

There are also a few other distinctive, but less numerous, neuronal cell types in the neocortex, among which are fusiform cells and horizontal cells of Cajal (Figure 8–2).

Fusiform cells, sometimes called **multiform cells**, are found only in layer VI (the deepest layer) of neocortex. They have a cigar- or fusiform-shaped cell body, with dendrites extending from both poles. These dendrites are branched but have few or no spines.

Horizontal cells of Cajal are relatively few in number and are located in the most superficial layer of the neocortex. Their dendrites extend laterally from the cell, parallel with the surface of the cerebral cortex.

B. Layers of Neocortex

The six layers of the neocortex, from the pial surface to the deep white matter, are as follows (Figure 8–3):

Layer I: The **molecular layer**, also called the **plexiform layer**, is made up primarily of the dendritic and axonic arborizations of other cells. Its only cell bodies are the few horizontal cells of Cajal.

Layer II: The **external granular layer** contains primarily stellate, or granular, cells, although there are always at least a few pyramidal cells.

Layer III: The **external pyramidal layer** is dominated by pyramidal cells. It also contains a fair number of stellate cells. Both of these cell types receive most of their information from **association fibers** and **commissural fibers**—that is, from other portions of the cerebral cortex.

Association fibers are those whose cell bodies are elsewhere in the same cerebral hemisphere. Commissural fibers are those whose cell bodies are in the opposite cerebral hemisphere.

Layer IV: The **internal granular layer**, as its name implies, is composed primarily of stellate, or granular, cells. It also contains a few pyramidal cells. It receives most of the terminal endings of **thalamo-cortical axons**.

Layer V: The **internal pyramidal layer** contains the largest pyramidal cells and a few stellate, or granular cells. The axons of its pyramidal cells form many of the **projection fibers** that go from the cerebral cortex to subcortical structures and to other cortical areas via either **association tracts** or the **corpus callosum**.

Layer VI: The **fusiform layer**, or **multiform layer**, is the deepest layer. It is immediately above the deep white matter of the cerebral cortex. The fusiform layer is characterized by fusiform cells, whose axons leave the cerebral cortex and project either to subcortical structures or to other areas of the cortex by way of association fibers in the deep white matter.

C. Classifying Neocortex by Extent of Pyramidal and Granular Layers

There is more than one way to classify a neocortex. In 1929, **Constantin von Economo** divided the human cerebral cortex into five major types of neocortex, based on the relative sizes of the populations of stellate and pyramidal neurons in each. Like Brodmann's, von Economo's taxonomy of neocortical organization has functional significance. His five classes are (Figure 8–3):

- *Agranular neocortex* is also known as motor cortex because it is the characteristic organization of the motor cortices. "Agranular" means that it contains few stellate (granular) cells and many pyramidal cells. Thus layers III and V are the dominant layers in this type of cortex.
- *Frontal neocortex* is found primarily in **association cortical areas**—specifically in the **frontal lobe anterior to the motor cortices**, and in the **superior parietal lobule** and **middle and inferior temporal gyri**. Although domi-

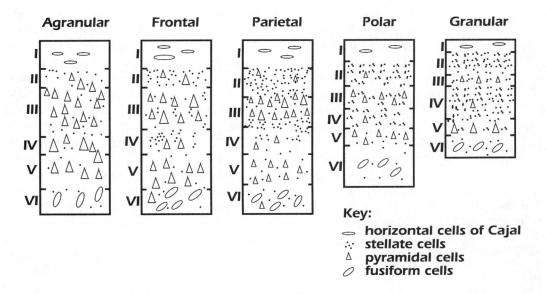

Figure 8–3. Types of neocortex as classified by von Economo.

nated by pyramidal cells, this cortex also contains a fair number of stellate cells.

- *Parietal neocortex* has an approximately equal distribution of pyramidal and stellate cells, and approximately equal thicknesses of all six neocortical layers. It is characteristic of some **association cortices** such as **Wernicke's area** and the **supramarginal** and **angular gyri**.
- *Polar neocortex* is found in the *inferior portion of the frontal lobe*, in an area known as the **orbital frontal cortex**, and in **areas 18 and 19**, the **association visual cortices**. It is a relatively thin neocortex containing fewer pyramidal cells and more stellate cells than parietal neocortex. Thus layers II and IV are more prominent than layers III and V in polar neocortex.
- *Granular neocortex*, also called **koniocortex**, is found in **primary sensory cortices**. This neocortex tends to be thin, with few pyramidal cells and numerous stellate cells. Layer IV is particularly prominent in the granular neocortices of **Brodmann's area 41 (auditory), area 2 (somatic sensory)**, and **area 17** along the **calcarine fissure (primary visual cortex)**.

D. Vertical Organization of Neocortex

The striking structural differences between the layers of the neocortex suggest a "horizontal" (i.e., parallel to the surface) organization. However, the functional organization of the neocortex at the neuronal level is not horizontal but vertical, or columnar (Figure 8–4). Axons extend into the neocortex and course vertically (i.e., at right angles to the surface of the neocortex) through its layers, making synaptic contacts with dendrites and cell bodies of neocortical neurons of different layers. Most of the synaptic terminals of these axons are on stellate cells of layers II and IV, although some synapse with dendrites of pyramidal cells, fusiform cells, and horizontal cells of Cajal of other layers. Both stellate cells and horizontal cells of Cajal are **Golgi II cells**. Their short axons arborize and synapse with pyramidal cells and fusiform cells of layers III, V, and VI, whose cell bodies are *This parallel coursing of afferent and efferent axons in a column helps to anatomically define these functional units.* just superficial or just deep to them. The pyramidal and fusiform neurons are the **Golgi I** (i.e., projection) neurons of the neocortex. Their axons exit the neocortex in a trajectory paralleling that of entering axons; then they enter the white matter deep to the neocortex. These pyramidal and fusiform axons synapse with either subcortical neurons or cortical neurons in other parts of the cerebral cortex.

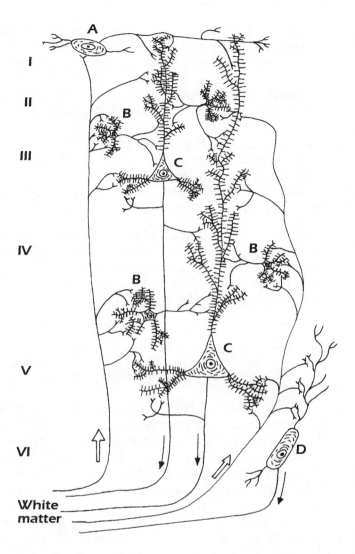

Figure 8–4. Schematic diagram of a few of the neurons and their synaptic relations in a single column of neocortex. Open arrows indicate axons entering the column. Closed arrows are the projection cell axons carrying information out of the column. Roman numerals are neocortical layers. **A** is a horizontal cell of Cajal; **B**s are stellate cells; **C**s are pyramidal cells; and **D** is a fusiform cell.

The neocortex consists of an extremely large number of columns of neurons. Each column includes neurons of all six neocortical layers and makes up a functional unit. Columns communicate with one another by way of **association pathways** formed when axons of projection fibers of one column enter first the white matter deep to the neocortex and then another cortical column. If the columns are close together, these projection fibers are **short association pathways**; if the columns are from distant parts of the cortex, the projection fibers are **long association pathways**. Each column processes neural information coming to it with its **local circuit (Golgi II) neurons** and sends the processed information out via its **projection (Golgi I) neurons**.

As early as the beginning of the 20th century, **Santiago Ramón y Cajal** noted that the only unique feature he could find in the human cerebral cortex was that it contained proportionally many more Golgi II cells than the cerebral cortices of other mammals.

Since then, the research of many workers has made it evident that this greater density of Golgi II cells is the anatomical basis for the extremely sophisticated neuronal processing done by the human neocortex. It may well hold the key to the phenomenon we call consciousness.

Summary

About 10% of the cerebral cortex is allocortex; the remaining 90% is neocortex, which contains few neuronal cell types. Most numerous are pyramidal cells (projection neurons) and stellate cells (local circuit neurons). In addition, there are horizontal cells of Cajal in the superficial layer and fusiform cells in the deepest layer.

Brodmann's numbering system defines structurally and functionally distinct areas of the cerebral cortex.

Neocortex has six layers, distinguished by the neurons they contain: from the surface these layers are:

- I—molecular layer
- II—external granular layer
- III—external pyramidal layer
- IV—internal granular layer
- V—internal pyramidal layer
- VI—fusiform layer.

Von Economo divided the human neocortex into five types based on the thickness of the different layers.

> Functionally, however, the neocortex is organized not in layers but in columns of cells. Each column includes all six neocortical layers. In any column, the neurons have similar functions.

II. AUDITORY PROCESSING OF SPEECH AND THEORIES OF SPEECH PERCEPTION

A. Auditory Processing of Speech

The neural messages the neocortex receives from the medial geniculate body must contain enough of the right kind of information to be decoded for the process we call speech perception to occur. Before considering the cerebrum's role in **speech perception**, therefore, we will consider how speech stimuli are processed in the **cochlea** and **subcortical auditory structures**.

Speech, like all other sounds, has three parameters: **frequency**, **intensity**, and **duration**. The cochlea, acting much like a sound spectrograph, analyzes speech for these three parameters and transduces them into patterns of nerve impulses. Therefore the **cochlear nuclei** receive a code of action potentials that contains both spectral and temporal representations of speech sounds.

Throughout the central auditory system, frequency information is represented in **tonotopic organizations**. The importance of frequency for speech perception lies not in the absolute frequencies of any utterance, which vary greatly from speaker to speaker, but in temporal changes of frequencies and in differences in frequency bands. These features are constant across speakers and carry important information for identifying both **phonetic** and **prosodic** aspects of speech. For example, both **formant transitions** and **glides** contain frequency sweeps that define **vowels**. Furthermore, both **stop consonants** and **fricatives** have distinct frequency representations. Frequency information is also important in perceiving prosody—both **stress** and **intonation patterns**.

Phonemes are the elementary features of speech. Prosody refers to patterns of rhythm, stress, and intonation of speech.

Duration of speech sounds also varies greatly across speakers and even for an individual speaker. However, certain durations are independent of speakers and provide essential cues to speech comprehension. For example, voiced and unvoiced consonant-vowel pairs, such as *pa* and *ba*, are distinguished solely by the times between the stop consonant and the beginning of voicing; these times differ only by milliseconds. Duration is also an important variable in understanding the prosodic element of stress.

Intensity of speech sounds also varies from speaker to speaker and in the same speaker. However, intensity changes in an utterance provide essential information for understanding both the stress and intonation patterns of prosody.

Therefore, the information coded in spiral ganglion neurons entering the brainstem contains the rudimentary information needed for speech perception. This information is significantly refined (i.e., processed) in the nuclei of the auditory brainstem:

- The **bushy cells** of AVCN retain and relay the frequency, duration, and intensity information.
- The **superior olivary neurons**, which have binaural input, add the dimension of sound localization and send the information on to the inferior colliculus.
- The **octopus cells** of PVCN code for frequency bands, rather than pure tones as eighth nerve fibers do. These frequency bands are approximately equal to the frequency bands of vowel formants. This significant information is sent to the inferior colliculus.
- The **multipolar neurons** of VCN code for stimulus onset, change, and termination—information that is essential to the perception of formant transitions, glides, and stop consonants—and pass it on to the inferior colliculus.
- The **inferior colliculus** receives all this highly sophisticated information, integrates it, and sends it to the **medial geniculate body**. Both the inferior colliculus and the medial geniculate body contain neurons that respond to frequency modulation (i.e., sweeps) and to intensity modulation.

So before speech information reaches the cerebral cortex, it has already undergone a great deal of processing in the cochlea and subcortical auditory centers. As sophisticated as that processing is, however, it is not sufficient by itself to explain speech perception. It cannot explain, for example, how we determine **segmentation** confusions which are resolvable only by connotation and context—how, for example, we distinguish "I scream" from "ice cream." It also does not explain how the brain understands many aspects of speaker variability, such as articulation differences and co-articulation, within utterances. The explanation of these extremely important aspects of speech perception must therefore lie in what happens in the cerebral cortex.

The cochlea's and brain's analyses of the neural coding of speech up to and then within the cortex is called **"bottom-up" analysis**. By contrast, the analysis of the use of stored cerebral knowledge to enhance and constrain speech perception is called **"top-down" analysis**. A complete explanation of speech perception involves both bottom-up and top-down analyses.

As you will see, most speech perception theories involve both bottom-up and top-down strategies.

Before we examine the role of the cerebrum in speech perception, let us have a brief look at the general theories of speech perception.

B. Theories of Speech Perception

Several theories have been proposed to explain speech perception, as happens with most poorly understood phenomena. None of the theories has been proven; all are consistent with at least some experimental data. They are particularly important to researchers who can formulate experiments to test their validity.

The ***psychoacoustic theory*** assumes that the spectral and temporal characteristics of the speech signal are the sources of speech information. This information is processed by the auditory system (bottom-up) with the help of cognitive (cerebral) processes (top-down). Speech information is processed similarly to the way nonspeech auditory information is processed by both humans and nonhuman mammals.

The ***direct realist theory*** assumes that the articulatory gestures—the positions and movements of the vocal tract, including lips and tongue, during speech—are the sources of speech information. These articulatory gestures are perceived not only by their spectral and temporal acoustic cues but also by vision, and, if one touches the lips, also by tactile cues. The information is processed by the sensory systems (bottom-up) with the help of cognitive (cerebral) processes (top-down). As in the psychoacoustic theory, speech information is processed similarly to nonspeech information in both humans and nonhumans.

This undefined language program is evidently in neither Broca's nor Wernicke's area. However, it interacts with both those defined areas.

The **motor theory** assumes that speech perception is mediated by an innate neural program that prepares infants to learn language in general. According to this theory, infants learn and then perceive language by comparing what they hear with this genetically determined neural program. The top-down analysis of comparisons is the critical aspect; the bottom-up processing of sounds or gestures is not emphasized. The mechanisms of speech perception are considered to be unique to humans.

Magnet refers to the idea that, during infant development, sounds similar to the key sounds of the native language are perceptually drawn to those key sounds, as if by a magnet, and absorbed by them so that the discriminations between them are lost.

The **native language magnet theory** does not attempt to explain all of speech perception but offers an explanation of how infants learn their native language. The theory, which is consistent with a considerable amount of experimental data, assumes that the infant can discriminate sounds very early in life. As they hear speech, they learn which discriminations are important in their native language and which are not. They master the important discriminations during infancy and lose the unimportant discriminations, even though the latter may be important in other languages.

The diversity of these theories of speech perception underlines our limited understanding of the subject. However, despite our limited understanding of *how* speech perception happens, we have considerable information about *where* in the cerebrum it occurs. The remainder of this chapter deals with this subject.

Summary

The cochlea processes sounds (including speech sounds) by frequency, intensity, and duration. Each of these parameters contains information that is necessary for understanding speech, including phonetics and prosody. Subcortical auditory processing further refines this information, coding for frequency bands, onset and termination, sound source, frequency modulation, and intensity modulation. Therefore, when speech information reaches the cerebral cortex, it is already sophisticated.

Various theories have been advanced to explain speech perception. These theories include the psychoacoustic theory, the direct realist theory, the motor theory, and the native language magnet theory. Each theory is more conceptual than mechanical and is consistent with certain experimental data. However, none is proven and none fully explains speech perception.

III. NEOCORTICAL ORGANIZATION AND SPEECH PERCEPTION

Specific auditory information necessary for understanding speech is projected from the ventral division of the medial geniculate body, through the sublenticular internal capsule, and into the primary auditory cortices (areas 41 and 42), which lie on the **transverse gyri of Heschl** on the superior surface of the temporal lobe (Figure 8–5). There are from one to three of these gyri, and often a different number on the left and right sides of the same brain. As far as is known, there is no functional significance to either the number or the frequent asymmetry.

In fact, some brains have one transverse gyrus on the left and three on the right.

Structurally, **area 41** is a **granular neocortex** (i.e., **koniocortex**) with few pyramidal cells and a thick layer IV of stellate cells. Based on the organization of its layers, area 41 is

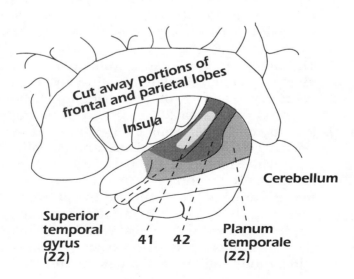

Figure 8–5. Details of the organization of primary auditory cortices (areas 41, 42) on two transverse gyri of Heschl and association cortex (area 22) on the planum temporale and posterior two-thirds of the superior temporal gyrus.

There are several tonotopic organizations of neurons in the transverse gyri of Heschl—not just one.

primary auditory cortex, and it receives most of its input from the ventral division of the medial geniculate body. The ventral division of the medial geniculate body also projects axons heavily to **area 42**, which encompasses the rest of the cortex of the transverse gyri of Heschl and may also extend slightly onto the planum temporale for distances that vary from brain to brain. Area 42 therefore is also primary auditory cortex; however, for reasons that are not understood, it has the neuronal structure of a **parietal (association) cortex** with all six layers about equally developed.

Auditory information that is received and processed by areas 41 and 42 (primary auditory cortex) is passed on to **area 22** (the posterior two-thirds of the superior temporal gyrus and the planum temporale) by short association fibers. Thus area 22 is an **association auditory cortex**.

In two-thirds of human brains, area 22 is larger on the left side than on the right. In the other one-third, area 22 is either the same size on both right and left sides, or larger on the right. This asymmetry may be the structural basis for the fact that speech perception and comprehension are dependent on the left area 22 in over 90% of people (i.e., all right-handed people and most left-handed people). Most of the remaining left-handed people have speech dependence in the right area 22, but a few can perceive and comprehend speech in both right and left areas 22. The area 22 that comprehends speech is named Wernicke's area whether it is on the right side, the left side, or both sides.

The largest tract emanating from area 22 is the **arcuate fasciculus**, a long association pathway that starts in the temporal lobe (Figure 8–6). It is made up of axons of projection neurons from area 22 and from some adjacent temporal lobe areas. These axons course around the posterior superior edge of the lateral fissure and extend anteriorly in the deep white matter of the parietal lobe and into the frontal lobe, finally terminating in the **area triangularis (Brodmann's areas 44 and 45)** and the **prefrontal cortex**. However, not all fibers of the arcuate fasciculus go directly to the frontal cortex. Many make synaptic connections for further integration in the neocortical columns of the **angular** and **supramarginal gyri, areas 39 and 40**.

These gyri (areas 39 and 40) also receive extensive sensory information from other sensory cortical areas, including

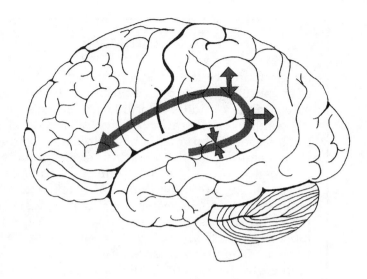

Figure 8–6. Lateral view of the brain showing the course of the arcuate fasciculus and its interaction with the angular and supramarginal gyri.

vision (from **areas 17, 18, and 19**) and somesthesia (from **areas 3, 1, and 2** and the **superior parietal lobule**). Thus the supramarginal and angular gyri are multimodality association cortices capable of integrating what is heard, what is seen, and what is felt. They are therefore of great importance in reading and writing.

The output fibers from the angular and supramarginal gyri (areas 39 and 40) join the arcuate fasciculus, traveling anteriorly in the deep white matter to carry information to the areas 44 and 45 in the frontal lobe, where motor processing of speech information occurs. Areas 44 and 45, like area 22, are functionally asymmetric, although not structurally asymmetric. Motor processing of speech occurs in the left areas 44 and 45 in over 90% of people and in all those who are right-handed. Most left-handed people processes motor speech in the left areas 44 and 45; some left-handers process motor speech in the right areas 44 and 45, and a few do it in both right and left. The areas 44 and 45 that process motor speech, whether on the left, right, or both sides, are named **Broca's area**.

Language organization and the initiation of speech are covered in Chapter 9.

Summary

Information needed for speech perception enters the primary auditory cortex via the sublenticular internal capsule. Primary auditory cortex (Brodmann's areas 41 and 42) comprises the transverse gyri of Heschl. There is great anatomical variation in the number of transverse gyri. From primary auditory cortex, short association fibers project to area 22, which comprises the posterior two-thirds of the superior temporal gyrus and the planum temporale. In most people, the left area 22 is larger than the right; this asymmetry correlates with the fact that in most people left area 22 is necessary for speech comprehension. The arcuate fasciculus carries information from area 22 to the area triangularis (areas 44 and 45) and the prefrontal cortex. Along this pathway, the arcuate fasciculus interacts with the angular (area 39) and supramarginal (area 40) gyri. The left area triangularis is needed for proper expressive speech in all right-handed people and in most left-handed people.

CHAPTER 8 SUMMARY

The cerebral cortex, which is 90% neocortex and 10% allocortex, can be subdivided by any of three schemes:

- by Brodmann's numerical system;
- by the major lobes and their gyri;
- by von Economo's five types of neocortex, based on the thickness of the layers.

The major neuronal types in neocortex are pyramidal cells and stellate cells; minor neuronal types are horizontal cells of Cajal, in the most superficial layer, and fusiform cells, in the deepest layer.

There are six neocortical layers:

- I—molecular layer;
- II—external granular layer;
- III—external pyramidal layer;
- IV—internal granular layer;
- V—internal pyramidal layer;
- VI—fusiform layer.

The cochlea analyzes sounds for frequency, intensity, and duration, all of which contain important information for speech perception. The subcortical auditory system further analyzes speech signals for location, frequency bands and transitions, onset and termination, frequency modulation, and intensity modulation. Therefore the auditory cortex receives very sophisticated information about speech signals.

There are presently four major theories of speech perception:

- the psychoacoustic theory;
- the direct realist theory;
- the motor theory;
- the native language magnet theory.

All of these theories are consistent with various known characteristics of speech perception, but none are proven.

The transverse gyri of Heschl (areas 41 and 42) comprise the primary auditory cortices. Their anatomy varies among individuals and between sides of the brain in a given individual.

Area 22, made up of the posterior two-thirds of the superior temporal gyrus and the planum temporale, is an important association auditory cortex; in most people, it is larger on the left than on the right. In the speech dominant hemisphere (the left, in most people), this is Wernicke's area and is necessary for normal speech comprehension. The arcuate fasciculus connects area 22 with areas 44 and 45 (area triangularis) and with the prefrontal cortex. In the speech dominant hemisphere, area triangularis is Broca's area; it is necessary for normal expressive speech.

ADDITIONAL READING

Bellugi, V., Poizner, H., & Klima, E. S. (1989). Language, modality and the brain. *Trends in Neuroscience, 12,* 380–388.

Best, C. T. (in press). A direct realist view of cross-language speech perception. In W. Strange (Ed.), *Speech perception and linguistic experience: Theoretical and methodological issues in cross-language speech research.* Timornium, MD: York Press.

Damisco, A. R., & Geschwind, N. (1984). The neural basis of language. *Annual Review of Neuroscience, 7,* 127–147.

Geschwind, N. (1979). Specializations of the human brain. *Scientific American, 241,* 180–199.

Kolb, B., & Whishaw, I. Q. (1990). *Fundamentals of human neuropsychology* (3rd ed.). New York: Freeman.

Kuhl, P. K. (1994). Speech perception. In F. D. Minifie, (Ed.), *Introduction to communication sciences and disorders* (pp. 77–148). San Diego, CA: Singular Publishing Group.

Nauta, W. J. H., & Freitag, M. (1986). *Fundamental neuroanatomy.* New York: Freeman.

STUDY GUIDE

Answer each question with a brief paragraph

1. What is the primary structural difference between neocortex and allocortex?

2. Describe the Brodmann areas of particular interest to speech-language professionals.

3. What cell types are in the neocortex?

4. Describe the layers of neocortex.

5. What is a neocortical column?

6. Describe how frequency, intensity, and duration cues are important for speech perception.

7. Describe how brainstem auditory structures code for speech cues.

8. Briefly compare and contrast four theories of speech perception.

9. Describe the structural asymmetry of area 22 and what its possible functional significance is.

10. Describe the parts of and the functional role of the inferior parietal lobule.

Odd One Out

In each of the following questions, choose the item that does not "fit" with the other three; briefly explain what the other three have in common that the odd one lacks. There may be more than one correct answer.

1. ___ hippocampus

___ septal region

___ angular gyrus

___ parahippocampal gyrus

WHY?

2. ___ Brodmann's area 4

___ Brodmann's areas 3, 1, 2

___ Brodmann's area 6

___ Brodmann's areas 44, 45

WHY?

3. ___ pyramidal cells

___ stellate cells

___ fusiform cells

___ bushy cells

WHY?

4. ___ pyramidal cells

___ fusiform cells

___ Golgi type I
neurons

___ Golgi type II
neurons

WHY?

5. ___ frequency

___ intensity

___ duration

___ sound source

WHY?

6. ___ psychoacoustic
theory

___ direct realist
theory

___ motor theory

___ native language
magnet theory

WHY?

7. ___ transverse gyri
of Heschl

___ planum
temporale

___ angular gyrus

___ supramarginal
gyrus

WHY?

9

D. Webster
Neuroscience of Comm.
1995

THE ORGANIZATION OF LANGUAGE

Exposure to speech is necessary for a child to learn to speak. After that, however, the act of speaking depends on two decisions: whether to speak and what to say. Whether it's going to be a brief exclamation when you stub your toe, or a well thought out reply to a difficult question, your brain makes decisions before speech happens. These decisions—which can be influenced by perceptions, thoughts, memories, emotions, or any number of other things—are made in the prefrontal cortex.

I. PREFRONTAL CORTEX

The **prefrontal cortex** is the portion of the neocortex that lies in the frontal lobe, anterior to the motor areas (Figure 9–1). The motor areas include the **primary motor cortex**, the **premotor area**, the **supplementary motor area**, and **Broca's area**. The prefrontal cortex is larger in humans, relative to other portions of the brain, than in any other species.

The prefrontal cortex receives a great deal of information from other parts of the neocortex—parietal, frontal, and

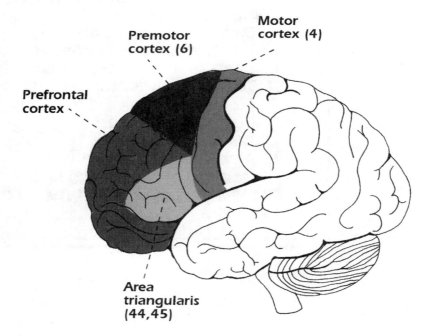

Figure 9–1. Lateral view of the brain showing the relationships of the prefrontal cortex and the motor areas of the lateral side of the frontal lobe.

temporal lobes—by way of the **arcuate fasciculus** and **superior longitudinal fasciculus**. In addition to immediate sensory information, these long association pathways also carry memories of past experiences and thoughts. In addition, by way of the **thalamus**, the prefrontal cortex receives information from the emotional centers of the brain—collectively called the **limbic lobe**.

The prefrontal cortex is thus uniquely qualified for decision making. Its importance is dramatically demonstrated by what happens to people who have an acquired loss in this part of the brain. In fact, most of the scientific data about how the prefrontal cortex functions has been gleaned from studies of people who had **prefrontal lobotomies**.

A prefrontal lobotomy surgically disconnects the prefrontal cortex from the rest of the brain. It was commonly performed earlier in the 20th century to relieve intractable pain and to treat people with severe violent and self-destructive psychiatric disorders. It is rarely performed today because, in most cases, pharmacology offers better treatments that are both effective and reversible (see "The First Studied Case . . .").

People with prefrontal lobotomies have no motor impairments and by most measures their intelligence is not affected; they can learn new things and remember old experiences. However, a prefrontal lobotomy does dramatically and irreversibly alter personality. People who have undergone this procedure lose the ability to make what we think of as rational decisions; they tend to act on impulse, without regard for later consequences; their behavior is often described as both irreverent and capricious; their speech contains much vulgarity; and they lose their respect for social conventions. Because they are not only irresponsible but also frequently offensive to many people, they are usually unable to hold jobs. However, they are harmless and less irritable than they probably were before. People who had the procedure because of excruciating, intractable pain report that the pain is still there but no longer bothers them.

Decisions, decisions: we make them every day. When the alarm rings and you know you have an 8:00 A.M. class, you have to make a decision. The emotional part of your brain may say, "Go back to sleep; I don't want to go to class," but the rational part of your brain will probably warn you that there will be consequences if you miss that class. Your memories may also come into play: you may have acted

---

THE FIRST STUDIED CASE OF A PREFRONTAL LOBOTOMY

On September 13, 1848, Phineas P. Gage, then 25 years old and the foreman of a railroad crew, had an accident. He was drilling holes in granite to prepare for dynamiting for new railroad tracks. As he tamped down the dynamite, it exploded. The blast sent the tamping rod, 3 cm in diameter and fine-pointed, through the orbit of his left eye and up through the prefrontal region of his brain. It destroyed much of his prefrontal cortex and dissociated the remainder from the rest of his brain. Amazingly, he survived this injury and, under a physician's care, was nursed back to perfect health. He retained full use of his motor functions, language, memories, and intelligence.

However, his personality was permanently altered: "This man is no longer Phineas P. Gage," said his friends. He had been known as a responsible workman and a pillar of the community. Now he was irresponsible, irreverent, and capricious, and his speech became vulgar and offensive. He was finally fired from his job. He wandered around the country and eventually lived in San Francisco under the custody of his family, where he died in 1861. Although no autopsy was performed, his skull was later recovered and bilateral damage to the prefrontal cortex was confirmed.

---

irresponsibly in the past and suffered consequences. So you probably decide, even if you do not feel like it, to get up and go to class.

But, if you had had a prefrontal lobotomy, you would have no dilemma here: if you did not feel like going to class, you would simply turn off the alarm and go back to sleep.

Among other decisions made in the prefrontal cortex are when and how to use language. Thus, although this portion of the brain has nothing to do with our understanding of language, it is important in our speech behavior.

Summary

The prefrontal cortex receives integrated information from sensory cortical areas, memory stores, and emotional areas of the brain (limbic lobe). The prefrontal cortex is where conscious decisions are made, including whether or not to speak.

II. LIMBIC LOBE: EMOTIONAL REPRESENTATION IN THE BRAIN

5 structures

Emotions are represented in various portions of the forebrain; these portions are collectively referred to as the **limbic lobe**. Of particular importance are:

- a portion of the deep temporal lobe called the **amygdala**;
- the **cingulate gyrus** just above the corpus callosum on the medial aspect of the brain;
- the **parahippocampal gyrus** of the medial temporal lobe;
- the **hippocampus**, bulging into the lateral ventricle in the temporal lobe;
- the **septal area** just under the genu of the corpus callosum;
- and a few smaller portions of the forebrain (Figures 9–2, 9–3).

Emotion plays an important role in the prosody of speech.

Note that all cortical areas of the limbic lobe are allocortex.

In experimental animals, electrical stimulation or surgical lesions of these structures result in behavioral changes—for example, showing fear, preparing to attack, or becoming very placid—that are specific to the area being stimulated. In humans we would call these emotional changes.

feeding
flight
fight
fear
Rep.

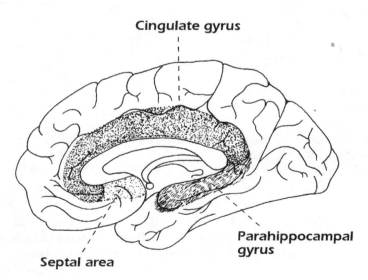

Cingulate gyrus

Parahippocampal gyrus

Septal area

Figure 9–2. Medial view of the right cerebrum after removal of the brainstem and cerebellum. Note how the cerebral cortices of the limbic lobe form a rim (limbus) around the corpus callosum and brainstem.

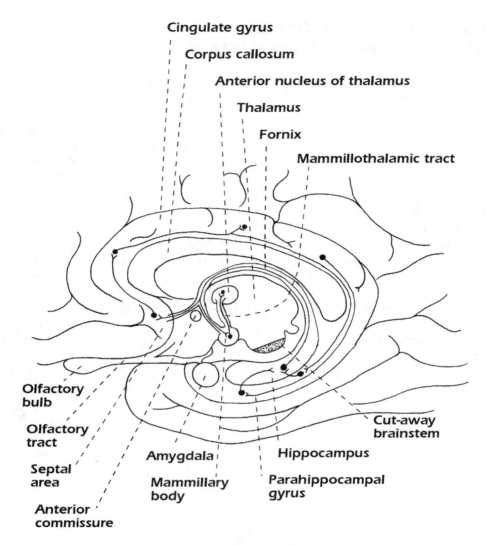

Cingulate gyrus

Corpus callosum

Anterior nucleus of thalamus

Thalamus

Fornix

Mammillothalamic tract

Olfactory
bulb

Olfactory
tract

Septal
area

Anterior
commissure

Amygdala

Mammillary
body

Hippocampus

Parahippocampal
gyrus

Cut-away
brainstem

Figure 9–3. Medial view of the right hemisphere with a dissection of the temporal lobe to expose the amygdala and hippocampus, and with a dissection of the thalamus to show the fornix and anterior nucleus of the thalamus. The brainstem and cerebellum have been cut away.

The neuronal circuitry of the limbic lobe is complex. The **amygdala** receives input from the **parahippocampal gyrus**, the **olfactory system**, the **hypothalamus**, and various thalamic nuclei. Fibers from the amygdala project to the **septal area**, the **parahippocampal gyrus**, and the **dorsal medial nucleus of the thalamus**. The primary projection of the dorsal medial nucleus of the thalamus is to the prefrontal cortex where, you will recall, decisions are made.

The **septal area** has reciprocal connections with the **cingulate gyrus** which, in turn, has reciprocal connections with the **parahippocampal gyrus**. The parahippocampal gyrus projects axons to the **hippocampus** which, in turn, projects axons via the **fornix** to both the septal area and the **mammillary bodies**. The axons of the mammillary bodies project to the **anterior nucleus of the thalamus** via the **mammillothalamic tract**. The **anterior nucleus of the thalamus** projects axons to the **cingulate gyrus** (Figures 9–2 and 9–3).

This complex circuitry of the limbic lobe is the neuronal basis for our equally complex emotions (see box "The First Scientific Demonstrations...").

Some patients with extensive damage in the language portions of the brain—particularly in both Broca's and Wernicke's areas—are virtually speechless, yet the limbic lobe has enough speech capability to cause very emotional single words to be spoken. Thus, to the dismay of relatives and friends, the only speech of some patients with this type of damage consists of emotional, often scatalogical, words uttered with great energy.

You will shortly learn about global aphasias. The utterances of people with global aphasias are probably expressions from the limbic lobe, particularly the cingulate gyrus.

Summary

The limbic lobe comprises diverse portions of the forebrain that are primarily concerned with emotions. These various limbic lobe structures project to the prefrontal cortex via the anterior nucleus of the thalamus and the dorsal medial nucleus of the thalamus.

III. NEUROBIOLOGY OF MEMORY

We take **memory** for granted. We recall things that happened recently as well as things that happened in the past; we rarely think about the mechanisms of memory, or whether there are discrete locations in the brain that specifically subserve memory.

An analysis of memory indicates that it is a complex process. First, the memory must be *acquired*—that is, it must be laid

THE FIRST SCIENTIFIC DEMONSTRATIONS OF EMOTIONAL CENTERS OF THE BRAIN

In 1937, James Papez, a neuroanatomist, described the brain circuitry of what is now known as the limbic lobe, which involves several structures including the cingulate gyrus, the parahippocampal gyrus, the hippocampus, the fornix, the mammillary bodies of the hypothalamus, and the anterior nucleus of the thalamus. Based on the anatomical connections he described, he suggested that these structures could be involved in the affective or emotional behavior of animals—including people.

In the same year—1937—a neuropsychiatrist, Heinrick Klüver, and a neurosurgeon, Paul Busy, described the effects of deep, bilateral temporal lobe resections on a group of fierce male macaque monkeys that could not be safely handled. Following the temporal lobe resections, which destroyed most of the structures Papez had described as important for emotion, the behavior of these monkeys changed dramatically. They became placid and tame and could be handled easily. They showed repeated curiosity even about objects that had previously induced fear; they handled such objects, put them in their mouths, and picked them up for re-examination as if they had not already done so. They also showed hypersexual behavior.

The combination of the anatomical studies by Papez and the behavioral studies of Klüver and Busy were the first demonstrations of emotional centers in the brain.

Studies with experimental animals suggest that acquisition, storage, and retrieval are distinct neural events: one or more can occur independently of the others.

However, damage to other cortical areas, or even to the cerebellum, can also cause memory loss.

down somewhere in the brain. Then it must be *stored* in a relatively permanent manner. Finally it must be *retrieved* at a later time.

During the 20th century, experiments with both humans and animals have led to an appreciation of some of these memory mechanisms and their locations in the brain. We know from these studies that after bilateral loss of the **hippocampus** (Figure 9–3)—that allocortical structure deep in the temporal lobe that bulges into the lateral ventricle—both short-term memory and the ability to learn new things are lost. In the few cases of people with bilateral hippocampal loss, it has not affected their intelligence, their ability to use language or speech, or their ability to recall old memories. It has prevented them from acquiring new memories. These people recognize family and old friends, but not someone they met just a few minutes earlier. Thus it appears that the ability to lay down new, short-term memories lies in the hippocampus.

The most dramatic losses of long-term memories result from lesions in the middle and inferior gyri of the temporal lobe. The role of these neocortical regions in the retention of long-term memories appears to be quite important, although difficult to define specifically.

Although it is recognized that certain locations are important in memory, the neuronal mechanisms involved in laying down either short- or long-term memories are still elusive. Some theories suggest that phenomena such as repeated neuronal activation at synapses can lead toward either short-term memory acquisition in the hippocampus or long-term memory acquisition in other portions of the brain, particularly in the middle and inferior gyri of the temporal lobe.

We do know that there are abundant neuronal pathways from one part of the cerebral cortex to another through association fibers, and to the opposite hemisphere through the corpus callosum. Thus it is possible for information from the temporal lobes to go to other portions of the cerebral hemisphere—and presumably, therefore, to carry memory information.

Summary

Memory is a complex and poorly understood neurological event. It involves:

- memory acquisition
- memory storage
- memory retrieval.

Short term memory requires having at least one intact hippocampus. Although people with bilateral destruction of the hippocampus are unable to learn new things, they do retain old memories.

IV. BRAIN LESIONS AND SPEECH/LANGUAGE COMPREHENSION

Because **language** is a uniquely human attribute, its neurobiology can be studied only in humans. Much has been learned from studies of people who have brain lesions that

Some nonhuman animals— including many of our pets— certainly show some characteristics of language. But spoken and written language is unique to people.

do not directly affect speech or language. However, the most productive investigations have been of people who have acquired language deficits due to **focal brain lesions**. The most common type of focal brain lesion is caused by an occlusion of an artery that supplies blood to a specific portion of the brain. Because no bleeding occurs in this type of **stroke**, it does not damage adjacent parts of the brain that are supplied by other arteries. When the deficits that result from a focal brain lesion are specific to speech/language, they are called **aphasias**.

In the second half of the 19th century, **Paul Broca** and **Carl Wernicke** conducted landmark studies of patients with focal lesions in speech areas and did much to elucidate where human speech is localized in the brain. In the 20th century, **Norman Geschwind** and his colleagues have confirmed many of those old observations and have added new data from a wide variety of patients. The modern view of language organization in humans is greatly indebted both to the pioneering studies of Broca and Wernicke and to the 20th century observations and syntheses of Geschwind.

Some aspects of language, such as rhythm, are localized in the right hemispheres of people with left hemispheric dominance.

It was noted in the 19th century that most aphasias occurred after lesions to the **left cerebral hemisphere**. Many studies have now documented that in approximately 96% of aphasias the damage has been to the left hemisphere. From these studies the conclusion is drawn that all right-handed people and most left-handed people have language localized in their left hemispheres, which is therefore, in these people, called the **dominant hemisphere**. A few left-handed people have language in their right hemisphere (i.e., their right hemisphere is the dominant one), and a few have bilateral representation of language.

A. Damage to Broca's Area

Broca's area—areas 44 and 45—is the **area triangularis** in the frontal lobe of the dominant hemisphere (Figure 9–4). Occlusion of the branch of the **middle cerebral artery** supplying this area results in an **expressive aphasia** (also called **Broca's aphasia**). Speech is poorly articulated and produced with considerable effort. Because Broca's area lies close to the primary motor cortex in the precentral gyrus, many lesions that affect Broca's area also affect the adjacent primary motor cortex and produce paralyses or weakness on the right side of the body.

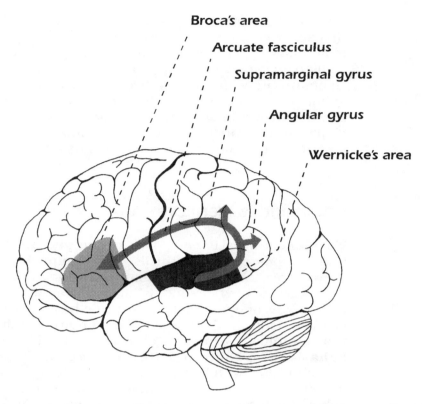

Broca's area

Arcuate fasciculus

Supramarginal gyrus

Angular gyrus

Wernicke's area

Figure 9–4. Lateral view of the left side of the brain showing Broca's and Wernicke's areas and the arcuate fasciculus.

However, whether or not there is paralysis or weakness, people with Broca's aphasias have problems not only with articulation but also with language. They are unable to produce correct sentences; particularly lacking are small grammatical words such as *and* and *if*. Thus the speech is linguistically impaired—that is, it is a specific language impairment, not just a paralysis. However, people with Broca's aphasia have good comprehension of both spoken and written language. It is therefore evident that Broca's area (areas 44 and 45) is critical to the expression of language.

B. Transcortical Motor Aphasia

If the cerebrum just anterior and dorsal to Broca's area is damaged, a **transcortical motor aphasia** results. This area is normally vascularized by terminal branches of the middle and anterior cerebral arteries. Areas vascularized by the terminal branches of arterial systems are called **fringe**

areas and are particularly vulnerable to strokes. Damage to this area disconnects Broca's area from the prefrontal, premotor, and supplementary motor cortices, but without seriously damaging them. Because Broca's area can no longer communicate with these cortices, spontaneous and conversational speech are severely impaired. However, because Broca's area is intact, there is remarkable retention of the ability to accurately *repeat* words, phrases, and even sentences. Speech comprehension is retained.

C. Damage to Wernicke's Area

Wernicke's area is composed of the **planum temporale** and the posterior two-thirds of the **superior temporal gyrus** (area 22) of the dominant hemisphere (Figure 9–4). As has been noted, area 22 is bilaterally an auditory association cortex and on the dominant side has specific language characteristics. If the branch of the **middle cerebral artery** that supplies Wernicke's area is occluded, a **receptive aphasia** (also called a **Wernicke's aphasia**) ensues. Although people with Wernicke's aphasia do not have hearing impairments (because the auditory areas of the other hemisphere are intact), they can no longer *understand* written or spoken language. Their own written and spoken language output is rapid and apparently effortless, but it contains little or no information. Rudimentary grammar is retained but the words do not give specific meaning.

Thus Wernicke's area is the neocortical area that is necessary for understanding language.

D. Transcortical Sensory Aphasia

If the cerebrum is damaged between Wernicke's area and the inferior parietal lobule (areas 39 and 40), a **transcortical sensory aphasia** results. This is a fringe area vascularized by terminal branches of the **middle** and **posterior cerebral arteries**. The damage disconnects Wernicke's area from the **angular** and **supramarginal gyri** without seriously damaging them. *Speech comprehension* is impaired; speech that is produced includes many *paraphrasias* and *word substitutions*. However, as in transcortical motor aphasia, the ability to *repeat* words, phrases, and sentences is retained.

E. Global Aphasia

When **Wernicke's area**, the **arcuate fasciculus**, *and* **Broca's area** are all damaged, the result is a **global aphasia**. These patients have profoundly impaired language—including their speaking, understanding, reading, and writing. Their spoken language is limited to a few isolated words, often with emotional content.

Recall that these utterances are probably from the limbic lobe.

F. Pure Word Deafness

Pure word deafness follows occlusion of the branch of the **middle cerebral artery** that supplies the nerve fibers passing from the **medial geniculate body** to the **auditory cortex** of the dominant hemisphere. This occlusion also destroys the portion of the **corpus callosum** that connects one auditory cortex with the other. Such patients have audiologically intact hearing, because auditory information still comes by way of the other medial geniculate to the other auditory cortex. However, this auditory information cannot pass from one cerebral hemisphere to the other because of damage to the corpus callosum. Therefore these patients have *no comprehension* of spoken language: they are "deaf" to the meaning of the words they hear.

However, in the occipital lobe their visual cortices are intact and can pass visual information via association fibers and callosal fibers to the **angular gyrus** (area 39) and to the **supramarginal gyrus** (area 40) in the **inferior parietal lobule** of the dominant hemisphere. The inferior parietal lobule in turn sends association fibers to Wernicke's area, where language is understood. Thus, in people with pure word deafness, *language is retained* but the *ability to understand spoken language is lost*, because there is no way for the spoken language to get to the language comprehension center in the dominant cerebral hemisphere.

G. Conduction Aphasia

A **conduction aphasia** occurs when an occlusion of a branch of the **middle cerebral artery** causes destruction of the **arcuate fasciculus** in either the parietal or frontal lobe of the dominant hemisphere (Figure 9–4). Recall that it is the arcuate fasciculus that carries information from areas 22, 39, and 40 into the **frontal lobe**, including **prefrontal cortex** and **Broca's area**. People with damage to the arcuate fasciculus *can understand spoken and written language*. However, because language comprehension in Wernicke's area cannot reach Broca's area, this information cannot be passed to the areas that are critical to language expression. People with such lesions *cannot repeat* things they have just heard and understood. In fact, conversation with such a person is most difficult because what they say has no relation to what they have just heard.

H. Alexia without Agraphia

When both the **visual cortex** of the dominant hemisphere and the **splenium of the corpus callosum** are destroyed, the ability to read is lost but the ability to write remains intact (Figure 9–5). Both of these portions of the brain are supplied by the **posterior cerebral artery**; occlusion of this artery in the dominant hemisphere causes this condition, which is called **alexia without agraphia**.

People with alexia without agraphia have unimpaired vision in their visual field on the dominant side, but at the cortical level their vision is confined to the occipital lobe on the nondominant side. Visual information in the nondominant cerebral hemisphere cannot pass to the dominant hemisphere because the fibers that would convey it, which pass through the splenium of the corpus callosum, have been destroyed. These patients have *normal language comprehension* and *normal speech production*, and they *can write*. But they *cannot read*—even what they themselves have written.

I. Isolation of the Speech Area

In extremely rare cases, a person will suffer damage to all or most of the neocortical areas surrounding the speech areas—**Broca's** and **Wernicke's areas**, the **supramarginal** and **angular gyri**, and the arcuate fasciculus—but no damage to those areas themselves. One such case, studied by Geschwind and his colleagues, was caused by carbon monoxide poisoning. The cerebral cortical damage was so

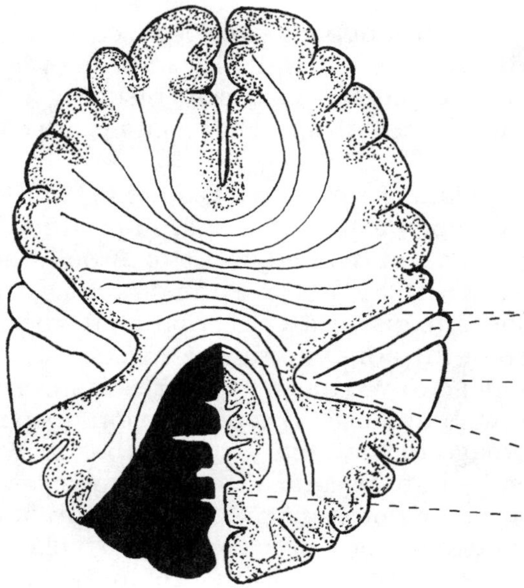

ANTERIOR

LEFT   RIGHT

POSTERIOR

Figure 9–5. Horizontal section of the cerebrum following occlusion of the left posterior cerebral artery causing destruction of the left visual cortex and the splenium of the corpus callosum. This damage results in alexia without agraphia.

extensive that the woman was incompetent to perform most tasks. However, in at least some cases she *could comprehend language.* She *could repeat perfectly phrases she heard.* She could also finish familiar phrases: for example, if the examiner said "Roses are red . . .," the patient would say "violets are blue, sugar is sweet and so are you." Even more remarkably, she was able to learn new material, probably because her left **hippocampus** was also intact. The radio in her hospital room was frequently turned on; she learned and sang songs that had not been written before the poisoning occurred.

Extreme cases like that outlined above demonstrate that language is organized in a restricted portion of the cerebral cortex—in 96% of people, on the left side—and that specific functions occur in discrete locations.

Summary

Speech and language are localized in the left cerebral hemisphere in all right-handed people and in most left-handed people. The deficits resulting from focal lesions that are specific to speech/language are called aphasias.

- Damage to Broca's area results in expressive aphasias with poorly articulated speech produced with effort.
- Damage to areas adjacent to Broca's area results in transcortical motor aphasias with impairment of spontaneous and conversational speech but retention of the ability to repeat speech.
- Damage to Wernicke's area results in receptive aphasia with impaired comprehension of speech.
- Damage to the area just posterior to Wernicke's area results in transcortical sensory aphasias with impaired speech comprehension but intact ability to repeat.
- Damage to both Broca's and Wernicke's areas results in global aphasias with profound impairment of all aspects of language.
- Damage to auditory radiation fibers and the adjacent corpus callosum fibers results in pure word deafness with no comprehension of spoken language but retained ability to read and write.
- Discrete destruction of the arcuate fasciculus results in conduction aphasias with loss of the ability to repeat language but retained language comprehension and expression.
- Damage to both the visual cortex of the dominant hemisphere and to the splenium of the corpus callosum results in alexia without agraphia; these patients can write but cannot read.
- Damage to most of the cortex of the dominant hemisphere except the specific speech structures isolates the speech area. Such a patient is greatly debilitated but can repeat phrases; language comprehension is extremely limited.

Broca's name is not included in this theory because he simply reported his observations without theorizing about them.

V. THE WERNICKE-GESCHWIND THEORY OF LANGUAGE

The most accepted theory of the neurobiology of language is the **Wernicke-Geschwind theory**. It is backed up by considerable data.

It proposes that language comprehension occurs when spoken language is passed from the medial geniculate body through the internal capsule up to primary auditory cortices—areas 41 and 42—and then by short association fibers to Wernicke's area. Written language is passed from the visual cortex to the supramarginal and angular gyri and to Wernicke's area.

Both spoken and written language are comprehended in Wernicke's area. The information is passed to the frontal lobes by the arcuate fasciculus, which carries information to both the prefrontal cortex and Broca's area. Decisions about whether to speak and what to say are made in the prefrontal cortex, and the encoding for expression of spoken language takes place in Broca's area, areas 44 and 45. The next stop on this "information superhighway" is the motor cortices, where speech production is initiated; this will be the subject of the next chapter.

Summary

The Wernicke-Geschwind theory of language is based on observations of specific impairments caused by diverse aphasias, each with its own focal lesions. The theory proposes that, in the dominant hemisphere, spoken information is passed from the primary auditory cortex to Wernicke's area for comprehension and written information is passed from the visual cortex to Wernicke's area, via the angular and supramarginal gyri, for comprehension. From Wernicke's area, the arcuate fasciculus carries the information to the prefrontal cortex and Broca's area. Coding for expressive speech occurs in Broca's area.

CHAPTER 9 SUMMARY

Decisions about when to speak and what to say are made in the prefrontal cortex. These decisions are determined by comparing the input from sensory systems, the limbic lobe, and sensory systems. Speech and language are localized in the left cerebral hemisphere of right-handed people and most left-handed people.

Focal lesions in the speech-dominant hemisphere can result in deficits that are specific to speech and language, named aphasias. The location of the focal lesion determines the type of aphasia that ensues. At least nine different aphasias, each resulting from a different lesion, are known.

The Wernicke-Geschwind theory of language is based on the location of the focal lesions in patients with specific aphasias. This theory proposes that speech/language information received from spoken language is passed by short association fibers from the primary auditory cortices to Wernicke's area for comprehension. Written language information is passed from the visual cortex by way of the angular and supramarginal gyri to Wernicke's area. Then the information is sent through the arcuate fasciculus to the prefrontal cortex and Broca's area. Expressive speech is coded in Broca's area.

ADDITIONAL READING

Damasio, H., Grabowski, T., Frank, R., Galaburda, A. M., & Damasio, A. R. (1994). The return of Phineas Gage: Clues about the brain from the skull of a famous patient. *Science, 264,* 1102–1105.

Fuster, J. M. (1989). *The prefrontal cortex: Anatomy, physiology, and neuropsychology of the frontal lobe* (2nd ed.). New York: Raven Press.

Geschwind, N. (1974). *Selected papers on language and the brain.* Boston: D. Reidel.

Isaacson, R. L. (1982). *The limbic system* (2nd ed.). New York: Plenum Press.

Squire, L. R. (1987). *Memory and the brain.* New York: Oxford University Press.

STUDY GUIDE

Answer each question with a brief paragraph

1. What are the effects of a prefrontal lobotomy on personality?

2. How does the prefrontal cortex affect language?

3. In what ways does the limbic lobe affect speech?

4. What is the role of the hippocampus in memory?

5. What is a focal brain lesion?

6. What is the speech dominant hemisphere and is it the same hemisphere in all people?

7. What blood vessels are involved in an expressive aphasia?

8. Describe the cause of a receptive aphasia and describe its effects on speech and language.

9. What aphasias do not damage the ability of a patient to repeat utterances that are heard?

10. Describe the neurological basic of pure word deafness.

11. Describe the Wernicke-Geschwind theory of language.

Odd One Out

In each of the following questions, choose the item that does not "fit" with the other three; briefly explain what the other three have in common that the odd one lacks. There may be more than one correct answer.

1. ____ primary motor cortex

   ____ premotor area

   ____ Broca's area

   ____ Wernicke's area

   WHY?

2. ____ arcuate fasciculus

   ____ superior longitudinal fasciculus

   ____ medial longitudinal fasciculus

   ____ internal capsule

   WHY?

3. ____ parahippocampal gyrus

   ____ subthalamus

   ____ olfactory system

   ____ hypothalamus

   WHY?

4. ___ storage

___ retrieval

___ short term

___ acquisition

WHY?

5. ___ Broca's aphasia

___ Wernicke's aphasia

___ global aphasia

___ transcortical motor aphasia

WHY?

6. ___ poor speech comprehension

___ paraphrasias

___ word substitutions

___ inability to repeat

WHY?

7. ___ no comprehension of spoken language

___ ability to read

___ ability to write

___ poor spoken language

WHY?

CHAPTER

10

SPEECH PRODUCTION

Once the decision to speak has been made in the prefrontal cortex and the information has been passed to Broca's area, the brain is ready for **speech production**. Speech is a motor task. Like other motor tasks—walking or manipulating items, for example—it begins in the central nervous system, passes through the peripheral nervous system, and results in movements of certain muscles which, in turn, move parts of the body.

I. PERIPHERAL SPEECH MECHANISM

Speech production uses many muscles in several parts of the body, including **respiratory**, **laryngeal**, **pharyngeal**, **soft palate**, **lingual**, **jaw**, and **lip** structures. Controlled, coordinated, synergistic movements of all these parts are necessary for normal speech. The disparate movements that occur during normal speech include the following, among others:

The complexities of these movements can be better appreciated if you consider that it takes 11 separate laryngeal muscles working together to adjust the vocal folds.

This is velopharyngeal closure. Controlled voice onset time determines whether these stop consonants are voiced or unvoiced.

- The respiratory rhythm changes so that more time is given to exhalation, when speech sounds occur, and less to inhalation.
- In the larynx, the **vocal folds** are approximated during **voiced sounds** so that the moving air column from the lungs can cause vocal fold vibrations. Conversely, they are separated during **unvoiced sounds** and during silent periods. Their mass and stiffness are precisely adjusted so that they vibrate at the appropriate frequencies during **vowel** production.
- The soft palate is raised against the back of the pharynx to avoid **nasal sounds** and lowered from the back of the pharynx to produce nasal sounds such as [m] and [n].
- The back of the tongue is raised against the palate for **stop consonants** [k] and [g].
- The tip of the tongue is raised to the alveolar ridge for stop consonants [t] and [d].
- The lips are pressed together for stop consonants [p] and [b].
- Constrictions are made in appropriate places along the vocal tract for **fricatives** such as [f] and [s].
- The volumes of the pharynx and oral cavity are altered to produce the resonances found in **vowel formants**.

It thus becomes clear that speaking even a simple sentence is rather like leading an orchestra: all of the complex movements of speech, like individual orchestra players, must work together with great temporal precision. Each must have precisely the correct degree of force, increasing or decreasing muscle tone (or musical volume) to the right degree and in the right sequence.

The process of speech production starts with information in Broca's area being passed, via short association fibers, to the motor cortices of the cerebral cortex.

Summary

The peripheral speech mechanism includes the respiratory muscles, lungs, larynx, pharynx, nasal cavity, palate, jaws, tongue, oral cavity, and lips. Energy for speech comes from the lungs, which set the approximated vocal folds into vibration during voiced sounds. Velopharyngeal closure eliminates nasal sounds. Stop consonants require closures at the palate, alveolar ridge, or lips. Specific constrictions of the vocal tract are required for fricatives. Supraglottal resonances are determined by the volumes of the pharynx and oral cavity. Speech production requires the coordinated activity of a large number of muscles.

II. MOTOR CORTICES

The **primary motor cortex** is **Brodmann's area 4**, which is comprised of the **precentral gyrus** and the anterior portion of the **paracentral lobule** on the medial surface of the cerebral hemisphere. It is an agranular cortex in which pyramidal cells predominate.

Primary motor cortex is made up of clusters of columns of neurons; each cluster of columns controls a single muscle of the body. The axons of the **pyramidal cells** in the primary motor cortex extend down through the internal capsule and go either to motor nuclei of the brainstem or to ventral horn cells of the spinal cord. In most of the body, axons from the left motor cortex cross the midline and go only to the motor nuclei of the opposite side of the spinal cord and brainstem. However, most muscles of the head and larynx have bilateral representation—that is, each motor cortex sends axons to the motor nuclei going to the head and laryngeal muscles on both right and left sides.

The "mapping out" of the way body parts are represented on the precentral gyrus produces a distorted representation of the whole body, which is called a homunculus.

The organization of neurons representing different muscles is very orderly. The muscles of the legs and feet are represented in the anterior portion of the paracentral lobule. The rest of the body is represented progressively along the precentral gyrus, from the midline down toward the lateral fissure: first hip, then abdomen, thorax, arms, hands, neck, and face. Body areas that have the most intricate musculature, and therefore the finest control, are represented by larger portions of the primary motor cortex than are areas with few and large muscles. Thus the hand has a larger representation and the thorax a smaller representation than size alone would indicate. Not surprisingly, the muscles of the larynx, soft palate, tongue, and lips have very large representations, reflecting the large number of small muscles that provide intricate control of speech.

The primary motor cortex is not the only cortical motor area of the brain. There are also the **premotor cortex (Brodmann's area 6)** anterior to the upper part of the precentral gyrus and the **supplementary motor cortex** on the medial surface of the frontal lobe. The premotor and supplementary motor cortices have a different organization than the primary motor cortex. Here *groups* of muscles, rather than individual muscles, are represented. Stimulation of the premotor or supplementary motor cortices results in contractions of *groups* of muscles. The premotor and supplementary motor cortices receive information from both Broca's area and association cortices of the superior and inferior parietal lobules. The premotor and supplementary motor cortices are important in programming movements that require complex sequences of muscles including speech. They pass their information on to the primary motor cortex.

Although the motor cortices contain a huge number of neurons and occupy a relatively large portion of the frontal lobe, their neuronal circuitry alone is not sufficient to direct the highly coordinated fine movements that characterize human behavior, including the extremely complex coordination of muscular groups necessary for speech. Before the motor cortices send their axons to the brainstem and spinal cord, they must send information to, and receive information from, two other large structures of the brain that assist in the fine control of voluntary movements. These structures are the **basal ganglia**, located in deep portions of the cerebral hemispheres, and the **cerebellum**, which is attached to the brainstem.

Summary

The primary motor cortex comprises the precentral gyrus and the anterior part of the paracentral lobule. Clusters of cortical columns control individual muscles in an extremely orderly manner. The other motor cortices—premotor cortex and supplementary motor cortex—are organized differently in that *groups* of muscles are controlled by the clusters of cortical columns.

III. BASAL GANGLIA

The **basal ganglia** are three large nuclei that lie deep in the cerebral hemispheres. Two of these nuclei—the **caudate** and the **putamen**—are functionally one nucleus that has been split in half by the anterior limb of the **internal capsule**. The caudate lies anterior and medial to the anterior limb of the internal capsule; the putamen lies posterior and lateral to it. Just deep to the putamen is the third basal ganglion, the **globus pallidus**. All three are large neuronal groups that participate in voluntary motor activity. The putamen and globus pallidus together appear as a single lens-shaped nucleus and the pair together is named the **lenticular nucleus**.

Together, the caudate and putamen are called the neostriatum.

Until the mid-20th century, the **amygdala** was also considered a basal ganglion. It was reclassified because studies showed that it functions quite differently than the others and that it is concerned with emotional activity—particularly arousal, rage, and fright.

The three basal ganglia—the caudate, the putamen, and the globus pallidus—have strong interactions with two other nuclei that participate in motor activity and must therefore be discussed along with the basal ganglia. These are the **subthalamic nucleus**, which is separated from the globus pallidus by the internal capsule, and the **substantia nigra**, a large midbrain nucleus lying in the deep portion of the cerebral peduncle.

Functionally speaking, therefore, there are really five basal ganglia (Figure 10–1):

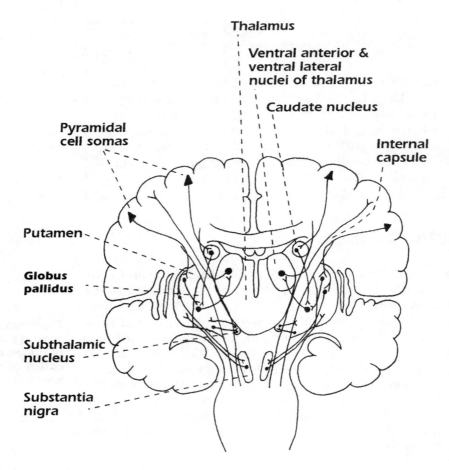

Figure 10–1. Schematic horizontal section showing the basic neuronal circuitry of the basal ganglia.

- **caudate**
- **putamen**
- **globus pallidus**
- **subthalamic nucleus**
- **substantia nigra**

A. Interactions of Basal Ganglia

Complex neuronal circuitry interconnects portions of the basal ganglia with one another and with the cerebral cortex by way of the thalamus. The motor cortices, and to a lesser extent other portions of the neocortex, send axons to the caudate and putamen. Both the caudate and putamen in turn send axons to synapse with neurons of the globus pallidus. The globus pallidus sends axons to thalamic nuclei called the **ventral lateral** and **ventral anterior nuclei of the thalamus**. These thalamic nuclei send axons via the internal capsule back up to the cerebral cortex, primarily to the motor cortices (Figure 10–1).

Although this circuitry does not include the subthalamic nucleus or the substantia nigra, both of these structures play important roles and have reciprocal interactions with the basal ganglia. The caudate and putamen both send axons to the substantia nigra, where there are complex interactions; then the substantia nigra sends axons back to the caudate and the putamen. Similarly, the globus pallidus sends axons to the subthalamic nucleus, which sends axons back to the globus pallidus (Figure 10–1).

B. Functions of Basal Ganglia

The best clues about the role of the basal ganglia in motor activity come from observations of the motor effects of lesions in various basal ganglia. Several motor diseases affect primarily one or another of the basal ganglia including the subthalamic nucleus and substantia nigra. All result in abnormal motor behavior, and more particularly, they all involve some involuntary movements—movements that are not willed and cannot be controlled (Table 10–1).

These basal ganglia diseases usually result from the loss of specific classes of neurons and their specific neurotransmitters. Because specific neurotransmitters are more concentrated in one nucleus than in others, these diseases are usually caused by damage to one specific nucleus.

Parkinson's disease, or **paralysis agitans**, is caused primarily by damage in the **substantia nigra**, although as this long-term disease progresses, other portions of basal ganglia and cerebral cortex are also gravely affected. Parkinson's disease is characterized by hypertonic rigidity of the muscles and by tremor of the extremities, particularly the hands. This tremor is prominent when a person is at rest but, at least in early stages, can be overcome when purposeful activity is undertaken. There is also a slowness of movement, called **bradykinesia**, and difficulty in both starting and ending movement. As the disease progresses, often over a 20-year period or more, all of these signs become more pronounced. They are accompanied by general dementia

Table 10–1
Diseases of the basal ganglia.

Syndrome	Nuclei Affected	Symptoms
Parkinson's disease	Substantia nigra; progresses to others	Hypertonic rigidity of muscles; tremor of extremities (especially hands), especially at rest; controllable in early stages during purposeful movements.
		Slow movement (bradykinesia); difficult to start/stop movements.
		Eventual general dementia; cerebral cortex degeneration; death.
Chorea ("dancing") diseases (e.g., Huntington's chorea)	Caudate and putamen; also some effect in globus pallidus	Jerky, irregular, rapid, purposeless movements, especially in distal part of extremities.
		Hypotonicity of muscles; prominent facial twitching.
Athetosis	Caudate and putamen	Muscle spasticity; involuntary, writhing, worm-like movements starting in proximal part of extremities.
Ballismus (same root as "ballistic")	Subthalamic nucleus; can be unilateral or bilateral	Hypertonicity; flailing, powerful, uncontrollable movements, especially of extremities. Arms and legs often broken by violent movements.

caused by cerebral cortex degeneration which worsens until death ensues.

The genetic mutation that causes Huntington's chorea has now been identified.

Chorea ("dancing") diseases are characterized by jerky, irregular, rapid, purposeless movements, particularly in the distal portion of the extremities. There is prominent facial twitching and general hypotonicity of the muscles. The primary damage in these diseases is to the **caudate** and the **putamen**, although the globus pallidus is also affected. The best known of these diseases is the genetic (inherited) disease, **Huntington's chorea**.

In **athetosis**, there is a characteristic spasticity of muscles with involuntary, writhing, worm-like movements originating in the proximal part of the extremities. The **caudate** and the **putamen** are the most affected nuclei.

In **ballismus** (same root as "ballistic"), there is a hypertonic motor condition with flailing, powerful, uncontrollable movements, particularly of the extremities. These movements can be so violent that people can break their arms or legs from hitting things. Ballismus is caused by destruction of the **subthalamic nucleus**; if the destruction is unilateral, only the muscles on the opposite side of the body are affected, but if there is bilateral destruction of the subthalamic nuclei, the ballistic movements are bilateral.

The disorder that follows unilateral disease of the subthalamic nucleus is called hemiballismus (hemi means half).

The basal ganglia receive information from and send information back to the cerebral cortex. They are high order modulators of motor activity; their primary motor role is to facilitate wanted movements and inhibit unwanted movements. One can think of the involuntary movements of basal ganglia diseases as activities that are normally suppressed, but which emerge when parts of the neural machinery—one or more portions of the basal ganglia—break down.

Summary

The basal ganglia process motor information, including speech information, to inhibit unwanted movements and facilitate wanted movements. The motor cortices project axons to the caudate and putamen. The caudate and putamen have reciprocal connections with the substantia nigra and project axons to the globus pallidus. The globus pallidus has reciprocal connections with the subthalamic nucleus and projects axons to the ventral anterior and ventral lateral nuclei of the thalamus. These thalamic nuclei then project the processed information back to the motor cortices. All diseases of the basal ganglia cause abnormal motor behaviors that involve involuntary movements.

IV. CEREBELLUM

While the motor cortices are interacting with the basal ganglia to inhibit unwanted movements and facilitate wanted movements, the cerebral cortex is interacting with the **cerebellum** to produce smooth, synergistic (i.e., coordinated)

The neuronal organization of the cerebellar cortex is totally different from that of the cerebral cortex. The cerebellar cortex has three layers and neuronal types not found in the cerebrum.

movements. From all parts of the cerebral cortex, and especially from the motor cortices, axons of **pyramidal cells** project down through the **internal capsule** and **cerebral peduncle** to synapse on the **pontine nuclei** in the ventral pons. Axons from these pontine nuclei project across the midline and, by way of the **middle cerebellar peduncle**, ascend into the cerebellum where they synapse directly on cerebellar cortical neurons (Figure 10–2).

The **cerebellar cortex** coordinates the activities of the muscles to be used. Axons of cerebellar cortical neurons project down into the deep portion of the cerebellum and make synaptic contacts with the group of nuclei collectively known as the deep cerebellar nuclei. Axons of **deep cerebellar nuclei** leave the cerebellum through the **superior cerebellar peduncle** and enter the midbrain tegmentum, where there is a massive crossing of fibers—those from the

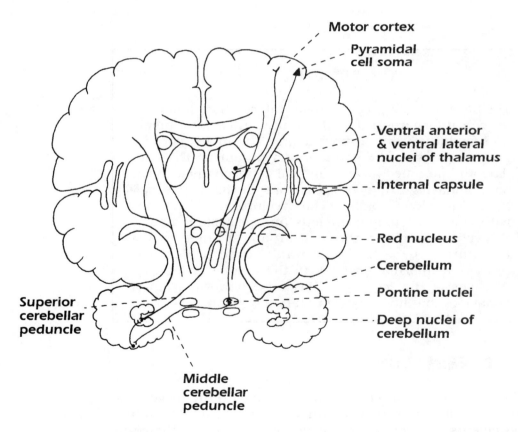

Motor cortex

Pyramidal cell soma

Ventral anterior & ventral lateral nuclei of thalamus

Internal capsule

Red nucleus

Cerebellum

Pontine nuclei

Deep nuclei of cerebellum

Superior cerebellar peduncle

Middle cerebellar peduncle

Figure 10–2. Schematic horizontal section showing the reciprocal neuronal circuitry between the cerebral cortex and the cerebellum.

right cerebellar hemisphere cross to the left and those from the left cerebellar hemisphere to the right. This is called the **decussation of the superior cerebellar peduncles**.

The axons—now back on the side of the brain where the information they carry originated—ascend into the diencephalon and synapse in the **ventral anterior** and **ventral lateral nuclei of the thalamus** (Figure 10–2). The axons of these two thalamic nuclei then project up through the internal capsule and back to the motor cortices. Thus there are reciprocal connections between cerebral cortex and cerebellum, just as there are between cerebral cortex and basal ganglia. If the cerebellum is damaged, coordination is lost: voluntary movements, which are usually smooth and coordinated, become uncoordinated and jerky. Furthermore, purposeful movements are accompanied by an uncontrollable tremor that is not present when the person is at rest.

The cerebellar tremor is called an intention tremor as opposed to the tremor that occurs at rest in patients with Parkinson's disease.

Summary

The cerebrum sends motor information to the cerebellum. It receives back from the cerebellum information that facilitates smooth, coordinated movements. Pyramidal cells of the motor cortices project axons to the pontine nuclei. Pontine nuclei neurons project axons across the midline to the opposite cerebellar cortex. The cerebellar cortex processes the information and sends it to the deep cerebellar nuclei. Information leaves the cerebellum via the superior cerebellar peduncle, which crosses the midline and projects to the ventral and anterior nuclei of the thalamus. These thalamic nuclei then project information back to the motor cortices. Cerebellar damage results in jerky volitional movements with an intention tremor.

V. UPPER MOTOR NEURONS

Once the motor cortices have interacted with the basal ganglia and cerebellum, their neurons send the appropriate instructions to motor nuclei of the brainstem and spinal cord. These projection pathways from cerebral cortex to motor nuclei are composed of **upper motor neurons**. The pathways to the spinal cord motor nuclei are somewhat different than those to brainstem motor nuclei.

A. Upper Motor Neurons to Spinal Cord

There are two upper motor neuron pathways to the spinal cord.

1. Corticospinal Pathway

Most of the axons of corticospinal neurons actually synapse with local circuit neurons which, in turn, synapse on the alpha and gamma motor neurons.

Many cortical motor neurons send their axons directly to spinal cord motor nuclei. These **corticospinal neurons** have long trajectories. They leave the motor cortices as part of the **corona radiata**, enter the **internal capsule** and then the **cerebral peduncles**, travel through the **ventral pons**, and finally emerge from the ventral pons as the **pyramidal tracts** on the anterior surface of the medulla. In the lower medulla, most of these pyramidal tract axons cross the midline as the **pyramidal decussation**; then they form the **lateral corticospinal tracts** of the lateral funiculus of the spinal cord. They finally terminate by synapsing with neurons of the anterior horn of the spinal cord. The pyramidal tract axons that do not cross in the pyramidal decussation continue into the spinal cord as the **anterior corticospinal tract**; they cross the midline in the spinal cord and synapse with neurons of the anterior horn of the spinal cord (Figure 10–3).

2. Corticorubrospinal Pathway

A second motor pathway from motor cortices to the spinal cord involves intermediate synapses in the **red nucleus** of the midbrain tegmentum and is called the **corticorubrospinal pathway**. Axons of cortical pyramidal cells leave the cortex as part of the **corona radiata**, enter the **internal capsule**, and then travel to the red nucleus and synapse there. Axons of red nucleus neurons then cross the midline as a decussation; they form the **rubrospinal tract**, which passes through the pontine tegmentum and the medulla to enter the lateral funiculus of the spinal cord. These axons finally terminate by synapsing on neurons of the anterior horn of the spinal cord (Figure 10–4).

3. Local Circuit Neurons

In the anterior horn of the spinal cord, axons of both the corticospinal and the corticorubrospinal pathways synapse

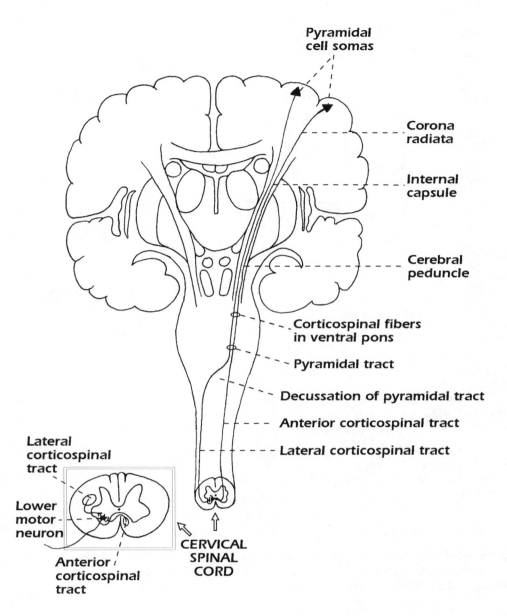

Figure 10-3. Schematic horizontal section showing the course of corticospinal neurons from the motor cortex to the spinal cord. Inset is a transverse section through the cervical spinal cord.

on small **local circuit neurons**. Axons of these neurons in turn synapse with the projection neurons of the anterior horn. Axons of anterior horn projection neurons pass out of the spinal cord to synapse with skeletal muscles.

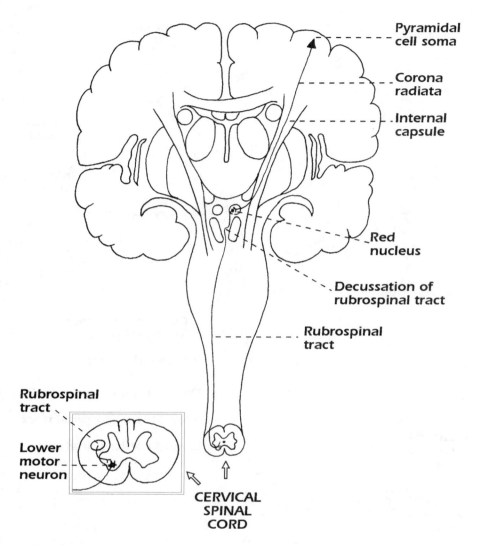

Figure 10–4. Schematic horizontal section showing the course of corticorubrospinal neurons from the motor cortex to the red nucleus and from the red nucleus to the spinal cord. Inset is a transverse section through the cervical spinal cord.

B. Upper Motor Neurons to Brainstem

The upper motor neuron pathway to the **brainstem motor nuclei** also originates in the motor cortices of the cerebrum. Axons of pyramidal cell neurons exit the cortex as part of the **corona radiata**, enter the **internal capsule**, and then travel to the brainstem motor nuclei. They are named **corticobulbar fibers** (the bulb is another name for the lower brainstem). Corticobulbar fibers from each cerebral cortex project to both right and left brainstem motor nuclei (in contrast to the corticospinal pathways, which are fully crossed) (Figure 10–5). Thus each motor cortex influences activity bilaterally in the brainstem. The only exception to this is that corticobulbar fibers to the upper part of the **facial nucleus** are all contralateral (to the opposite facial nucleus). Corticobulbar fibers, like corticospinal fibers, synapse on local circuit neurons in each brainstem motor nucleus; the axons of these local circuit neurons synapse on the projection neurons whose axons leave the brainstem to synapse on skeletal muscles.

C. Damage to Upper Motor Neurons

Damage to upper motor neurons results in what is called an **upper motor neuron syndrome**, in which volitional, but not nonvolitional, motor activity is impaired. The muscles affected by this syndrome, which have lost their input from the cerebral cortex, become hypertonic (spastic). Activity generated from noncerebral portions of the brain is still present, including reflexes, whose actions are exaggerated.

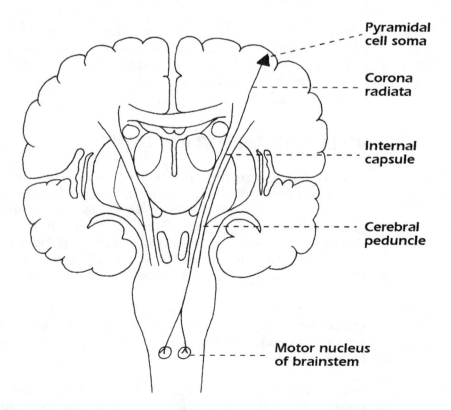

Figure 10–5. Schematic horizontal section showing the course of a corticobulbar neuron to brainstem motor nuclei.

You will learn more about dysarthrias and apraxias in Section VII of this chapter.

Because speech production is a volitional activity, it is affected by damage to the upper motor neurons projecting to the cranial nerve nuclei and the ventral horn cells that control respiration. The effects of such damage are most dramatic if the damage to the **primary motor cortex** is bilateral. There is a **spastic dysarthria** characterized by poor articulation, low pitch of voiced sounds, and a strained voice. Damage to either the **supplementary motor cortex** or the **premotor cortex** results in an **apraxia of speech** characterized by inconsistent but repeating errors in the sequencing of speech sounds.

Summary

The neurons that send motor information from the motor cortices to the motor nuclei of the brainstem and spinal cord are upper motor neurons. Corticospinal and corticorubrospinal pathways project to the spinal cord. Corticobulbar pathways project to the brainstem motor nuclei. Damage to upper motor neurons results in an upper motor neuron syndrome, in which muscles are spastic, reflexes are exaggerated, and volitional motor activity is impaired.

VI. LOWER MOTOR NEURONS

Lower motor neurons are defined as the neurons of the brainstem and spinal cord whose axons go directly to skeletal muscles. They include both **alpha motor neurons** and **gamma motor neurons**. They carry the final message through what is called the **final common pathway**—out of the central nervous system by way of peripheral nerves directly to the muscles that are to be activated (Figure 10–6).

The lower motor neurons important for speech and language are those that innervate the muscles of respiration and the muscles of the larynx, pharynx, palate, tongue, jaws, and face.

Spinal nerves innervate the muscles of respiration, whose control is vital to speech. Respiratory patterns must be altered so that more time is given to exhalation (when speech is produced) and less is given to inhalation (when it

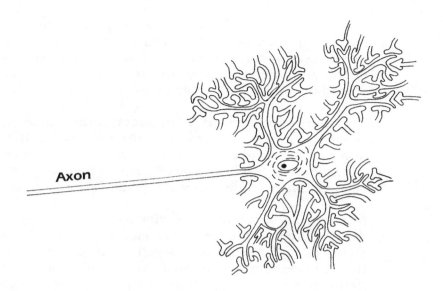

Axon

Figure 10–6. Diagram of a single lower motor neuron with hundreds of terminal boutons from the axons of other neurons synapsing on the dendrites, cell body, and axon of the lower motor neuron. The pattern of action potentials of the axon of the lower motor neuron depends on the sum of the excitatory and inhibitory activity of the neurons synapsing on it. For this reason the axons of the lower motor neurons form what is called the final common pathway.

is not). Moreover, loud speech requires stronger respiratory movements than soft speech.

Several brainstem motor nuclei are also involved in speech production. In the medulla, the **hypoglossal nucleus** contains lower motor neurons whose axons form **cranial nerve XII** (the **hypoglossal nerve**) to the tongue musculature. The **nucleus ambiguus** contains the lower motor neurons whose axons form **cranial nerves IX, X, and XI**—the **glossopharyngeal**, the **vagus**, and the **spinal accessory**. Spinal accessory fibers join the vagus nerve, travel as part of the vagus nerve, and then form the **superior and recurrent laryngeal nerves** which innervate the intrinsic muscles of the larynx. Vagus nerve fibers pass out to innervate the major muscles of the pharynx, except for the stylopharyngeus, which is innervated by the glossopharyngeal nerve. The vagus nerve also contains the lower motor neurons for the muscles of the palate—except for the tensor veli palatini, which is innervated by the **trigeminal nerve**.

The **facial nucleus**, located in the pons, is the brainstem motor nucleus for the muscles of facial expression; of this group, the perioral muscles are especially important for speech production and accurate articulation. The facial nerve lower motor neurons also innervate the posterior belly of the digastricus muscle, the stylohyoid muscle, and the stapedius muscle of the middle ear.

The **motor nucleus of V**, or **masticator nucleus**, is the brainstem motor nucleus of the trigeminal nerve. It sends its lower motor neurons to the muscles of mastication and to the anterior belly of the digastricus, the mylohoid, the tensor veli palatini, and the tensor tympani of the middle ear.

In short, all of the muscles that participate in speech production are activated by lower motor neurons of the brainstem and spinal cord. In speech, as in other motor activities, the results are far more devastating if lower motor neurons are damaged than if upper motor neurons are damaged. Partial damage of lower motor neurons to specific muscles causes weakness and fasciculations (muscle twitching). If lower motor neurons to a specific muscle are totally destroyed, that muscle becomes flaccid; it does not contract, it loses its reflexes, and in time it withers away. A **lower motor neuron syndrome** includes weakness or loss of muscle tone, reduced reflexes, and diminished overall activity of the affected muscles.

For speech production, damage to lower motor neurons results in a **flaccid dysarthria** characterized by poor articulation, breathiness, and hypernasality. The extent of the flaccid dysarthria depends on which lower motor neurons are affected and how extensively they are affected.

Summary

Lower motor neurons are the alpha and gamma motor neurons whose axons innervate, respectively, the extrafusal muscle cells and intrafusal muscle cells of the skeletal muscles. They constitute the final common pathway of motor activity. Total loss of lower motor neurons in a skeletal muscle results in flaccid paralysis with eventual muscle atrophy. Partial damage to lower motor neurons in a muscle results in weakness, reduced reflexes, and loss of tone.

VII. DYSARTHRIAS AND APRAXIAS

Diseases or traumatic injuries (including strokes) that damage the motor structures involved in speech production cause dysfunctions of speech. These dysfunctions do *not* affect speech perception, speech comprehension, language, or expressive coding in Broca's area. They are divided into two broad categories: **dysarthrias** and **apraxias**.

A. Dysarthrias

Dysarthrias are disharmonies of speech, which are often described by patients as difficulty in talking. There are different types, which are determined by the location of the damage in the motor speech system.

- **Flaccid dysarthria**, caused by damage to brainstem lower motor neurons or motor cranial nerves, is characterized by hypernasal speech, poor articulation, and a breathy voice.
- **Spastic dysarthria**, caused by damage to neurons of the primary motor cortex, is characterized by extremely poor articulation, a strained voice quality, and a low-pitched voice.
- **Ataxic dysarthria**, caused by damage to the cerebellum (particularly the vermis), is characterized by irregular, jerky speech and syllable repetitions.
- **Hypokinetic dysarthria**, caused by damage to the substantia nigra (as in Parkinsonism), is characterized by a weak voice with many hesitations intermixed with brief rushes of speech.
- **Hyperkinetic dysarthria**, caused by damage to the caudate and putamen (as in Huntington's chorea), is characterized by irregularities in the rate, pitch, and loudness of speech, frequent stoppages of speech, and tics.

B. Apraxias

Apraxias are inabilities or difficulties in performing complex volitional acts in which diverse muscles behave in a predetermined sequence. The muscles themselves are not paralyzed or even weak, and they perform less complex tasks normally. Because speech is a complex volitional act, it is not surprising that there are **apraxias of speech**.

They are caused by damage to the **premotor area** and particularly the **supplementary motor area**. The speech of such patients is "scrambled," containing many phoneme substitutions and distortions. It also tends to be "groping" and the patient has difficulty starting utterances. Errors are inconsistent: several attempts to say the same thing may all contain different errors.

Summary

The nature of a dysarthria depends on which of the following structures is damaged:

- primary motor cortical neurons
- lower motor neurons
- cerebellar neurons
- substantia nigra neurons
- caudate and putamen neurons.

Each of these dysarthrias results in difficulty in talking but in no problems with speech perception, speech comprehension, language, or expressive coding. Apraxias of speech result from damage to the supplementary and premotor cortical areas, which code for the sequencing of language. The problems caused by apraxias of speech include repetitions, difficulty selecting phonemes, and inconsistent speech errors.

CHAPTER 10 SUMMARY

The phenomenon of speech production is both complex and orderly. Once the appropriate motor cortices have received information from Broca's area as to what is to be said and how it is to be said, they interact with the basal ganglia to facilitate wanted movements and inhibit unwanted movements. The motor cortices also interact with the cerebellum to make the movements coordinated and smooth. Then the motor cortices send a pattern of nerve impulses through upper motor neurons to lower motor neurons; this selectively activates lower motor neurons whose axons go to the appropriate muscles to either increase or decrease their tone in a highly organized, coordinated manner. The pathway from the lower motor neurons to the skeletal muscles is called the final common pathway.

Thus the final common pathway to each muscle contains information from the motor cortices for volitional movements. It also contains all information from subcortical regions of the nervous system, such as reflexes and vestibular activity (Figure 10–6). Indeed, speech production is a complicated and sophisticated motor activity, well worth the time and effort devoted to its study. The true wonder is that it is usually performed so well.

ADDITIONAL READING

Albin, R. L., Young, A. B., & Penney, J. B. (1989). The functional anatomy of basal ganglia disorders. *Trends in Neuroscience, 12,* 366–375.

Bernstein, U. (1967). *The coordination and regulation of movements.* Oxford: Pergamon Press.

Ito, M. (1984). *The cerebellum and neural control.* New York: Raven Press.

STUDY GUIDE

Answer each question with a brief paragraph

1. Describe the movements needed to produce stop consonants.
2. What movements of the vocal tract are needed for vowel production?
3. Describe the organization of the primary motor cortex.
4. Describe the course of corticospinal neuron axons.
5. What functions do the basal ganglia serve?
6. Describe the various results following discrete lesions of the basal ganglia.
7. What is the role of the cerebellum in speech production?
8. Define the term *upper motor neuron*.
9. Compare and contrast upper motor neuron syndrome with lower motor neuron syndrome.
10. Define and compare dysarthria and apraxia.
11. What is the final common pathway?

Odd One Out

In each of the following questions, choose the item that does not "fit" with the other three; briefly explain what the other three have in common that the odd one lacks. There may be more than one correct answer.

1. ___ vocal fold vibrations

   ___ raising the soft palate

   ___ pressing the lips together

   ___ pressing the tongue tip to the palate

   WHY?

2. ___ precentral gyrus

   ___ premotor cortex

   ___ supplementary motor area

   ___ Broca's area

   WHY?

3. ___ caudate

   ___ putamen

   ___ amygdala

   ___ globus pallidus

   WHY?

4. ___ Parkinson's disease

   ___ aphasia

   ___ athetosis

   ___ ballismus

   WHY?

5. ___ internal capsule

   ___ cerebral peduncle

   ___ middle cerebellar peduncle

   ___ inferior cerebellar peduncle

   WHY?

6. ___ corticospinal neurons

   ___ corticorubro-spinal neurons

   ___ corticobulbar neurons

   ___ corticopontine neurons

   WHY?

7. ___ nucleus ambiguus

   ___ nucleus solitarius

   ___ facial nucleus

   ___ masticator nucleus

   WHY?

8. ___ alpha motor neuron

   ___ gamma motor neuron

   ___ lower motor neuron

   ___ upper motor neuron

   WHY?

INDEX

f = figure; *t* = table

A